The Ultimate Way to Vegetarian Re...

Enjoy your Diet with These Amazing and Effortless Recipes for Busy People

Skye Webb

© **Copyright 2021 - All rights reserved.**

The content contained within this book may not be reproduced, duplicated or transmitted without direct written permission from the author or the publisher.

Under no circumstances will any blame or legal responsibility be held against the publisher, or author, for any damages, reparation, or monetary loss due to the information contained within this book. Either directly or indirectly.

Legal Notice:

This book is copyright protected. This book is only for personal use. You cannot amend, distribute, sell, use, quote or paraphrase any part, or the content within this book, without the consent of the author or publisher.

Disclaimer Notice:

Please note the information contained within this document is for educational and entertainment purposes only. All effort has been executed to present accurate, up to date, and reliable, complete information. No warranties of any kind are declared or implied. Readers acknowledge that the author is not engaging in the rendering of legal, financial, medical or professional advice. The content within this book has been derived from various sources. Please consult a licensed professional before attempting any techniques outlined in this book.

By reading this document, the reader agrees that under no circumstances is the author responsible for any losses, direct or indirect, which are incurred as a result of the use of information contained within this document, including, but not limited to, — errors, omissions, or inaccuracies.

Table of contents

- Nori Snack Rolls 6
- Risotto Bites 8
- Jicama and Guacamole 10
- Curried Tofu "Egg Salad" Pitas 12
- Garden Patch Sandwiches On Multigrain Bread 14
- Garden Salad Wraps 16
- Black Sesame Wonton Chips 19
- Marinated Mushroom Wraps 21
- Tamari Toasted Almonds 24
- Avocado And Tempeh Bacon Wraps 26
- Kale Chips 28
- Tempeh-Pimiento Cheeze Ball 30
- Peppers and Hummus 32
- Deconstructed Hummus Pitas 34
- Savory Roasted Chickpeas 36
- Savory Seed Crackers 38
- Tomato and Basil Bruschetta 41
- Refried Bean And Salsa Quesadillas 43
- Tempeh Tantrum Burgers 45
- Sesame-Wonton Crisps 48
- Macadamia-Cashew Patties 51
- Garlic Tahini Spread 54
- Balsamic Pearl Onions Bowls 56
- Basil Rice Bowls 58
- Turmeric Peppers Platter 60
- Capers Dip 62
- Radish and Walnuts Dip 64
- Mushroom Cakes 66
- Cabbage Sticks 68
- Crispy Brussels Sprouts 70
- Arugula Dip 72
- Coconut Bites 74
- Basil Eggplant Tapenade 76
- Hot Eggplant and Broccoli Spread 78
- Almond and Pine Nuts Spread 80
- Coconut Cashew Dip 82
- Green Beans Dip 84
- Coriander Mint Chutney 86

SPICED OKRA BITES	88
ROSEMARY CHARD DIP	90
SPINACH AND CHARD HUMMUS	92
VEGGIE SPREAD	94
POMEGRANATE DIP	96
TOMATO AND WATERMELON BITES	98
BROWN BETTY BANANAS FOSTER.	100
BREAD & BUTTER PUDDING	103
CUSTARD BREAD PUDDING	106
WARM RUM BUTTER SPICED CIDER	108

Nori Snack Rolls

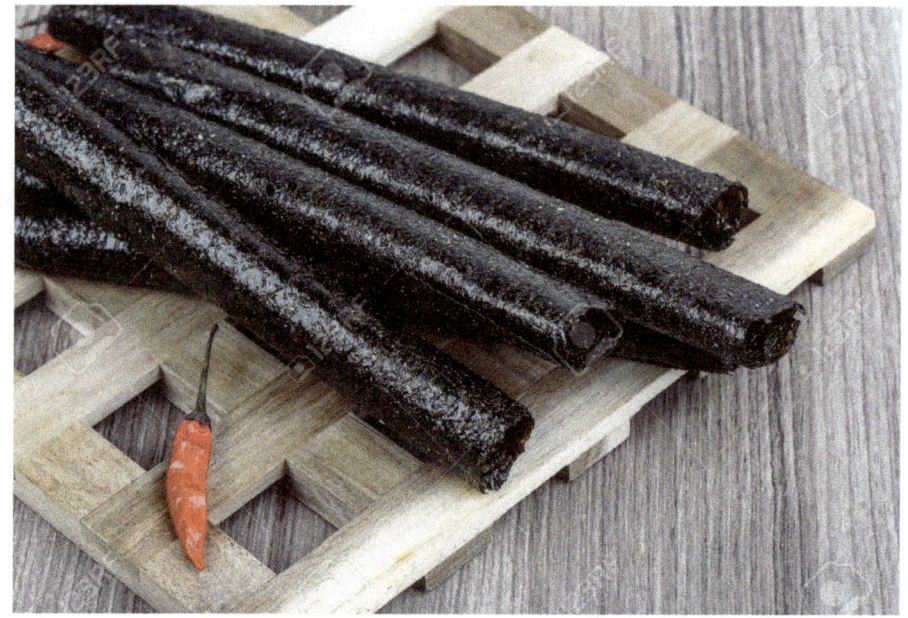

Preparation time: 5 minutes cooking time: 10 minutes servings: 4 rolls

Ingredients

2 tablespoons almond, cashew, peanut, or other nut butter

2 tablespoons tamari, or soy sauce

4 standard nori sheets 1 mushroom, sliced

1 tablespoon pickled ginger

½ cup grated carrots

Directions

1. Preheat the oven to 350°F.

2. Mix together the nut butter and tamari until smooth and very thick. Lay out a nori sheet, rough side up, the long way.

3. Spread a thin line of the tamari mixture on the far end of the nori sheet, from side to side. Lay the mushroom slices, ginger, and carrots in a line at the other end (the end closest to you).

4. Fold the vegetables inside the nori, rolling toward the tahini mixture, which will seal the roll. Repeat to make 4 rolls.

5. Put on a baking sheet and bake for 8 to 10 minutes, or until the rolls are slightly browned and crispy at the ends. Let the rolls cool for a few minutes, then slice each roll into 3 smaller pieces.

Nutrition (1 rollCalories: 79; Total fat: 5g; Carbs: 6g; Fiber: 2g; Protein: 4g

Risotto Bites

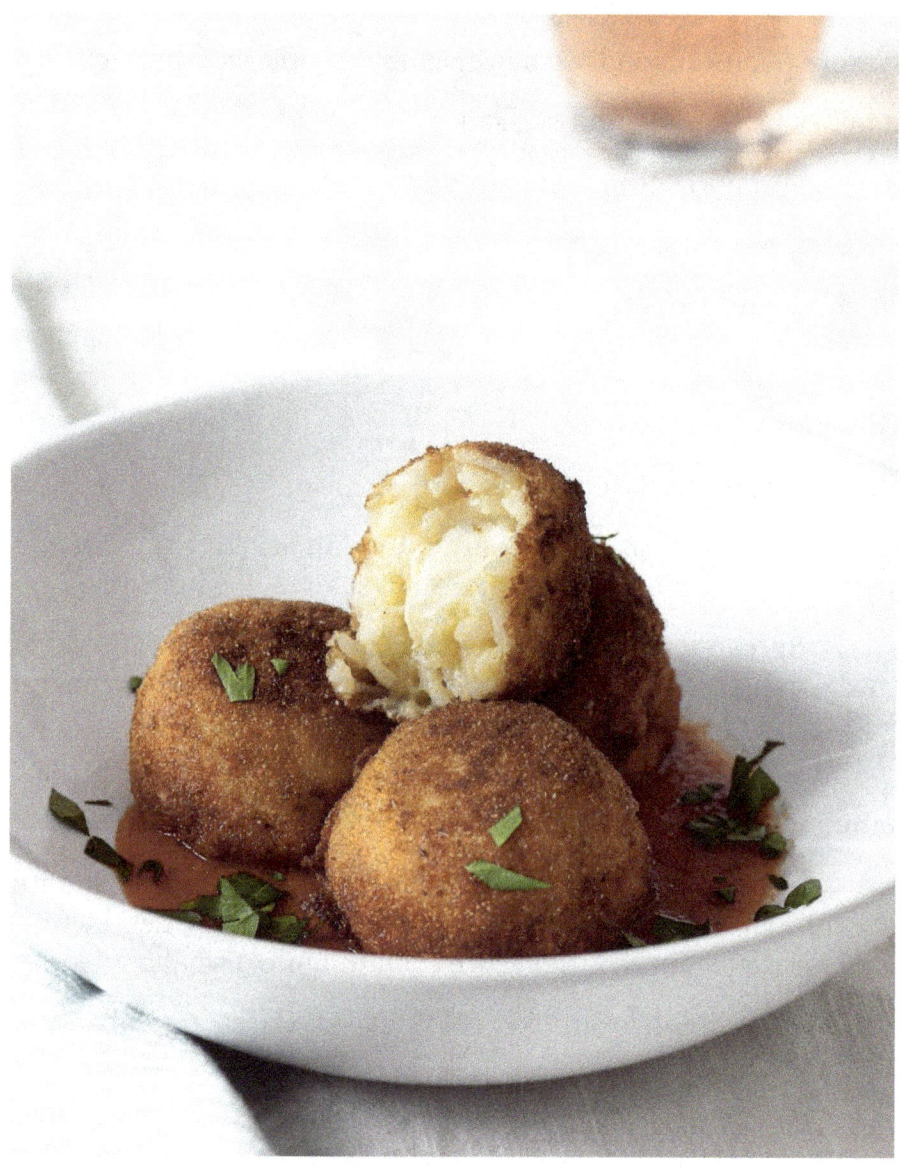

Preparation time: 15 minutes cooking time: 20 minutes servings: 12 bites

Ingredients

½ cup panko bread crumbs 1 teaspoon paprika

1	teaspoon chipotle powder or ground cayenne pepper

1½ cups cold Green Pea Risotto

Nonstick cooking spray

Directions

1.	Preheat the oven to 425°F.

2.	Line a baking sheet with parchment paper.

3.	On a large plate, combine the panko, paprika, and chipotle powder. Set aside.

4.	Roll 2 tablespoons of the risotto into a ball.

5.	Gently roll in the bread crumbs, and place on the prepared baking sheet. Repeat to make a total of 12 balls.

6.	Spritz the tops of the risotto bites with nonstick cooking spray and bake for 15 to 20 minutes, until they begin to brown. Cool completely before storing in a large airtight container in a single layer (add a piece of parchment paper for a second layeror in a plastic freezer bag.

Nutrition (6 bites): Calories: 100; Fat: 2g; Protein: 6g; Carbohydrates: 17g; Fiber: 5g; Sugar: 2g; Sodium: 165mg

Jicama and Guacamole

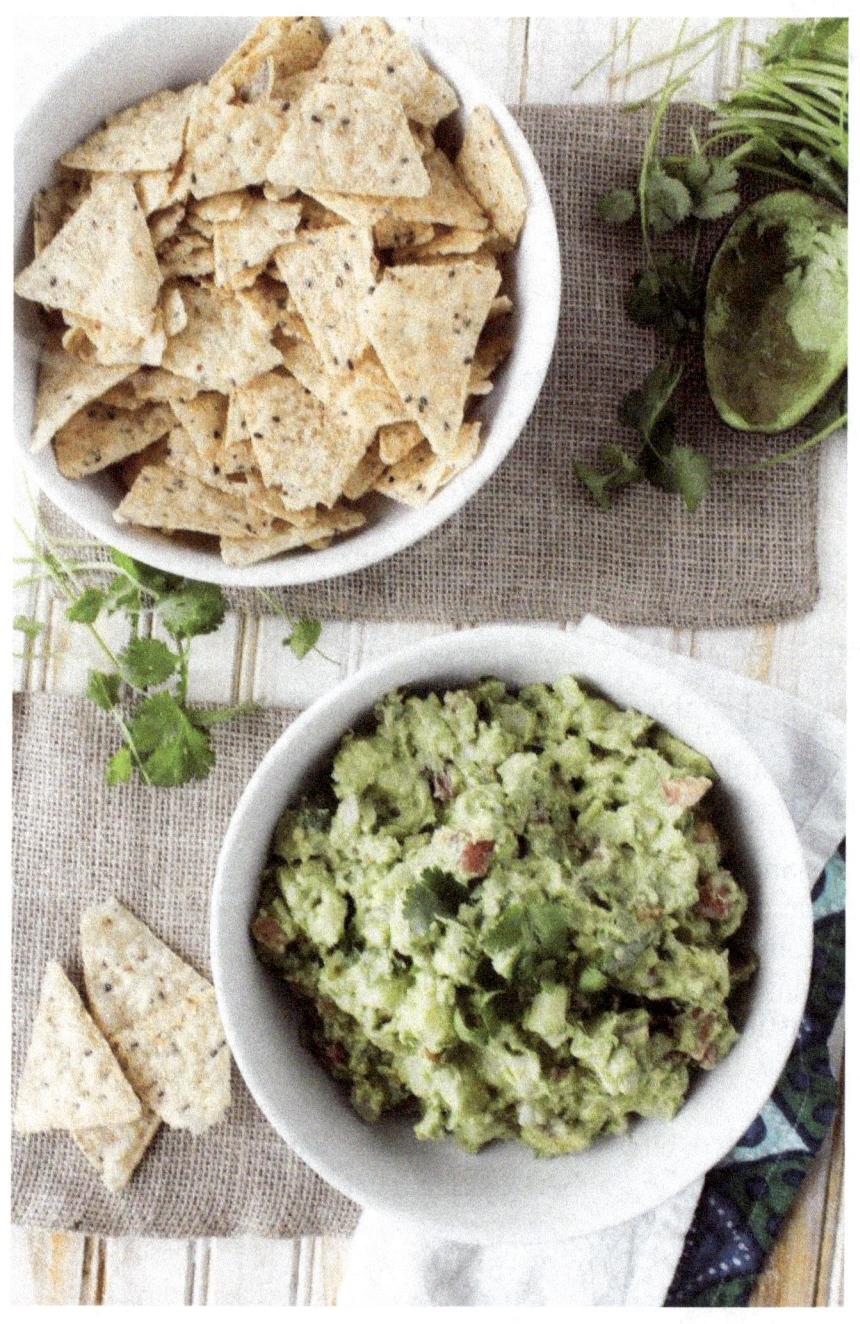

Preparation time: 15 minutes cooking time: 0 minutes servings: 4

Ingredients

juice of 1 lime, or 1 tablespoon prepared lime juice

2   hass avocados, peeled, pits removed, and cut into cubes

½ teaspoon sea salt

½ red onion, minced

1 garlic clove, minced

¼ cup chopped cilantro (optional

1 jicama bulb, peeled and cut into matchsticks

Directions

1.   In a medium bowl, squeeze the lime juice over the top of the avocado and sprinkle with salt.

2.   Lightly mash the avocado with a fork. Stir in the onion, garlic, and cilantro, if using.

3.   Serve with slices of jicama to dip in guacamole.

4.   To store, place plastic wrap over the bowl of guacamole and refrigerate. The guacamole will keep for about 2 days.

Curried Tofu "Egg Salad" Pitas

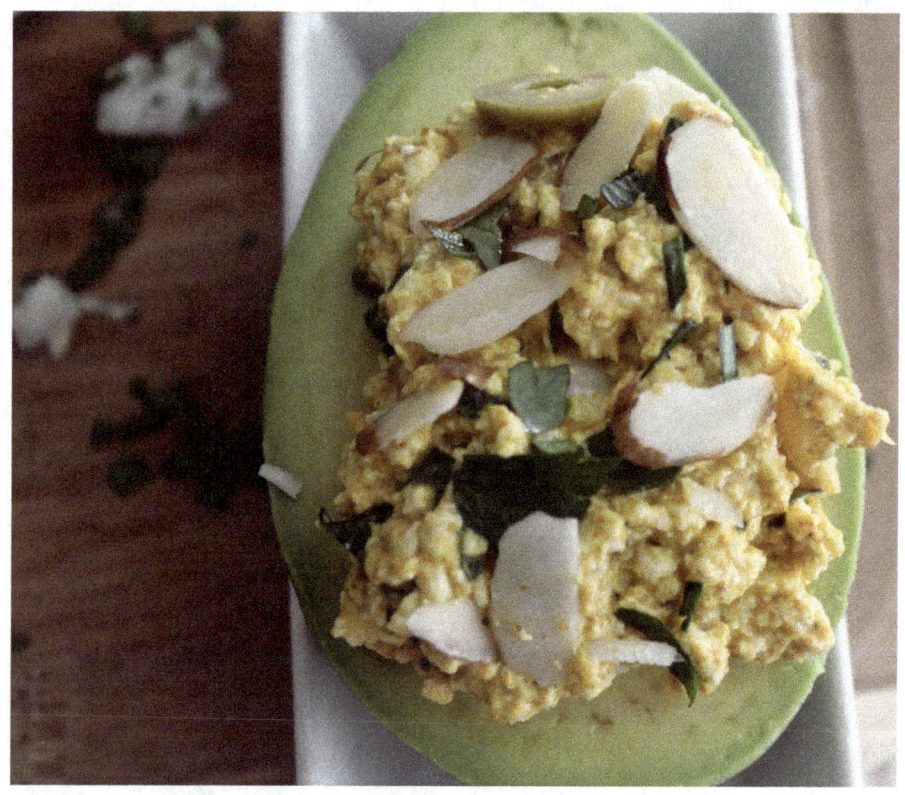

Preparation time: 15 minutes cooking time: 0 minutes servings: 4 sandwiches

Ingredients

1 pound extra-firm tofu, drained and patted dry

½ cup vegan mayonnaise, homemade or store-bought

¼ cup chopped mango chutney, homemade or store-bought

2 teaspoons Dijon mustard

1 tablespoon hot or mild curry powder

1 teaspoon salt

⅛ teaspoon ground cayenne

¾ cup shredded carrots

2 celery ribs, minced

¼ cup minced red onion

8 small Boston or other soft lettuce leaves

4 7-inchwhole wheat pita breads, halved

Directions

1. Crumble the tofu and place it in a large bowl. Add the mayonnaise, chutney, mustard, curry powder, salt, and cayenne, and stir well until thoroughly mixed.

2. Add the carrots, celery, and onion and stir to combine. Refrigerate for 30 minutes to allow the flavors to blend.

3. Tuck a lettuce leaf inside each pita pocket, spoon some tofu mixture on top of the lettuce, and serve.

Garden Patch Sandwiches On Multigrain Bread

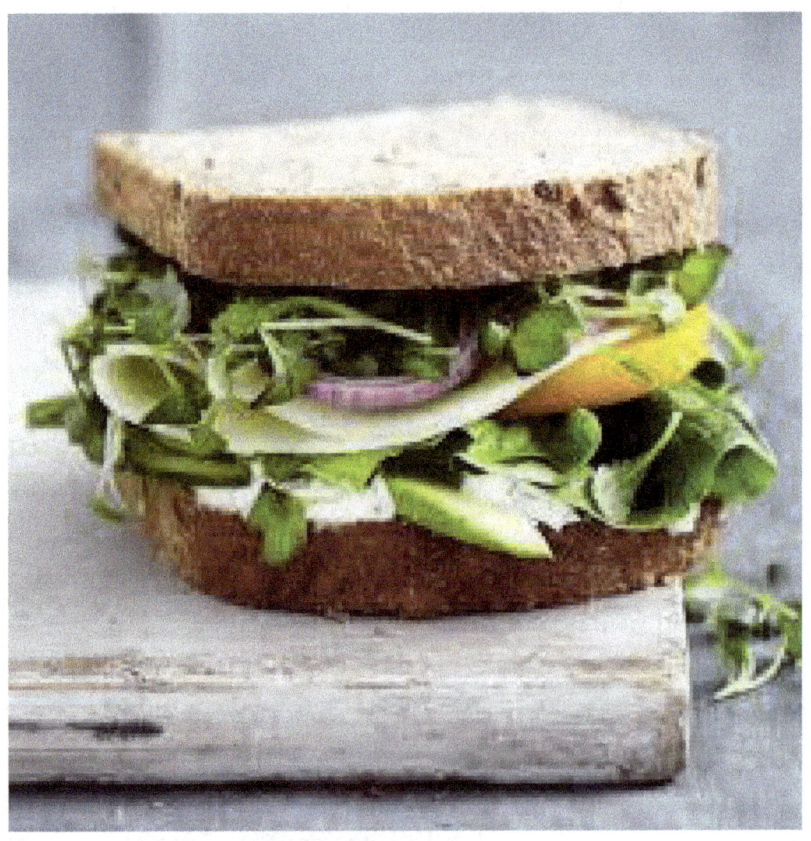

Preparation time: 15 minutes cooking time: 0 minutes servings: 4 sandwiches

Ingredients

1 pound extra-firm tofu, drained and patted dry

1 medium red bell pepper, finely chopped

1 celery rib, finely chopped

3 green onions, minced

1/4 cup shelled sunflower seeds

1/2 cup vegan mayonnaise, homemade or store-bought

1/2 teaspoon salt

1/2 teaspoon celery salt

1/4 teaspoon freshly ground black pepper

8 slices whole grain bread

4 (1/4-inch slices ripe tomato

4 lettuce leaves

Directions

1. Crumble the tofu and place it in a large bowl. Add the bell pepper, celery, green onions, and sunflower seeds. Stir in the mayonnaise, salt, celery salt, and pepper and mix until well combined.

2. Toast the bread, if desired. Spread the mixture evenly onto 4 slices of the bread. Top each with a tomato slice, lettuce leaf, and the remaining bread. Cut the sandwiches diagonally in half and serve.

Garden Salad Wraps

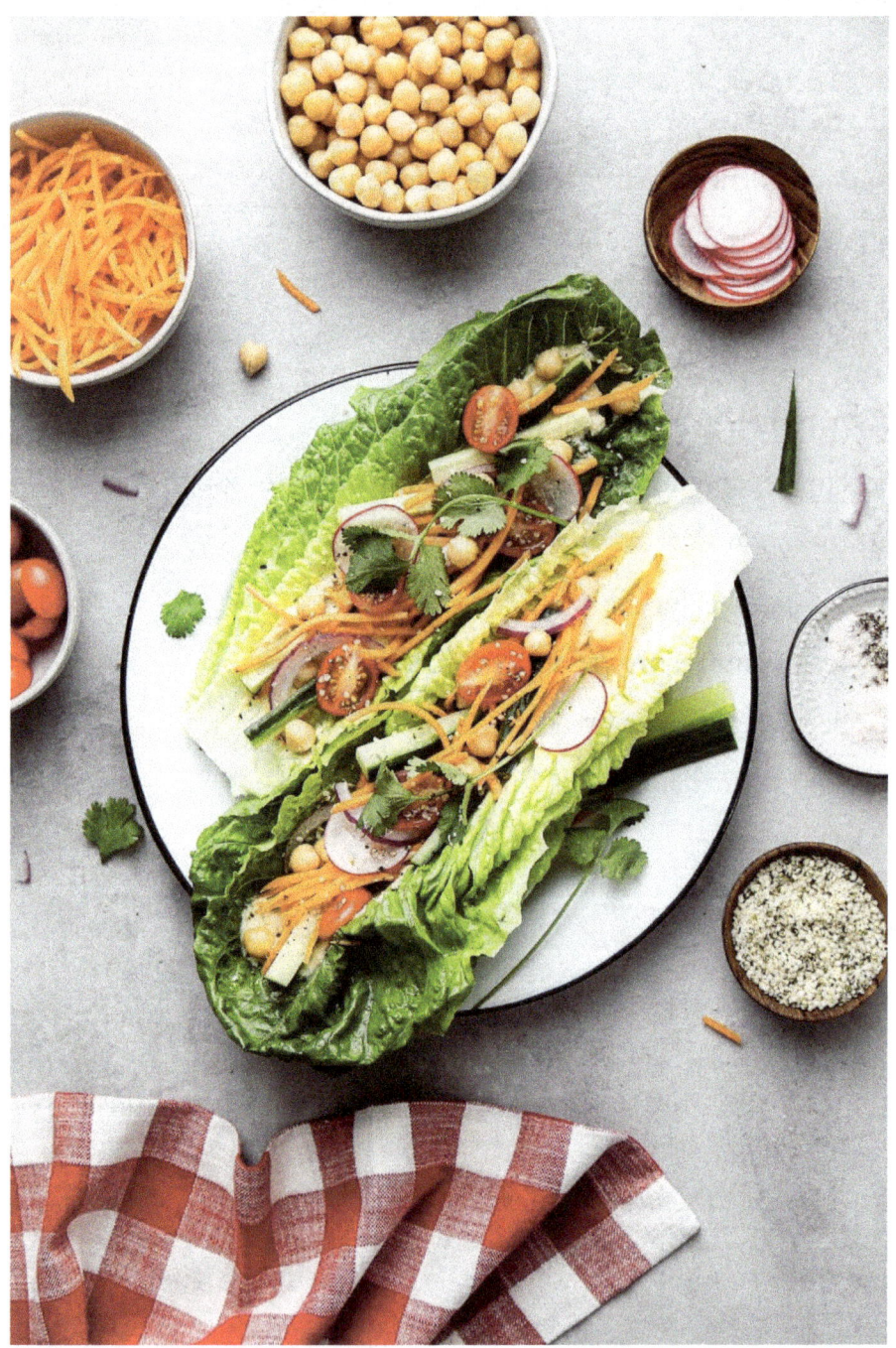

Preparation time: 15 minutes cooking time: 10 minutes servings: 4 wraps

Ingredients

6 tablespoons olive oil

1 pound extra-firm tofu, drained, patted dry, and cut into ½-inch strips

1 tablespoon soy sauce

¼ cup apple cider vinegar

1 teaspoon yellow or spicy brown mustard

½ teaspoon salt

¼ teaspoon freshly ground black pepper

3 cups shredded romaine lettuce

3 ripe Roma tomatoes, finely chopped

1 large carrot, shredded

1 medium English cucumber, peeled and chopped

⅓ cup minced red onion

¼ cup sliced pitted green olives

4 (10-inchwhole-grain flour tortillas or lavash flatbread

Directions

1.   In a large skillet, heat 2 tablespoons of the oil over medium heat. Add the tofu and cook until golden brown, about 10 minutes. Sprinkle with soy sauce and set aside to cool.

2.	In a small bowl, combine the vinegar, mustard, salt, and pepper with the remaining 4 tablespoons oil, stirring to blend well. Set aside.

3.	In a large bowl, combine the lettuce, tomatoes, carrot, cucumber, onion, and olives. Pour on the dressing and toss to coat.

4.	To assemble wraps, place 1 tortilla on a work surface and spread with about one-quarter of the salad. Place a few strips of tofu on the tortilla and roll up tightly. Slice in half

Black Sesame Wonton Chips

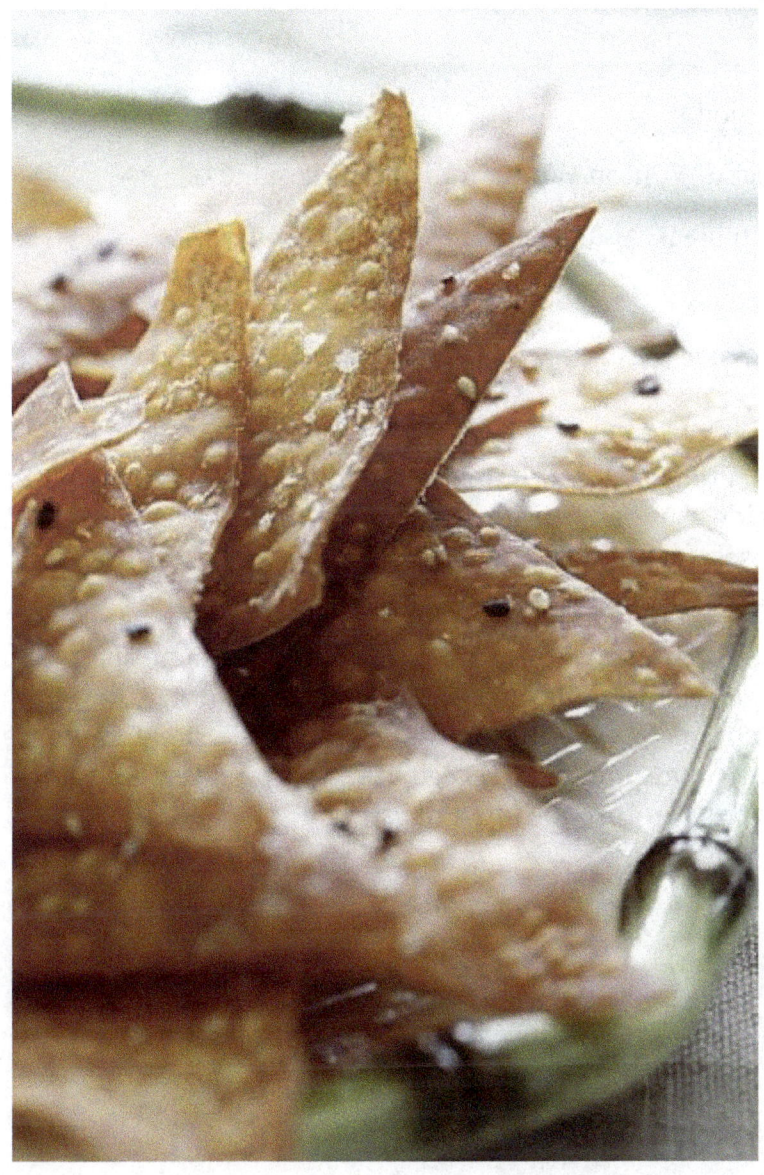

Preparation time: 5 minutes cooking time: 5 minutes servings: 24 chips

Ingredients

12 Vegan Wonton Wrappers Toasted sesame oil

1/3 cup black sesame seeds Salt

Directions

1. Preheat the oven to 450°F. Lightly oil a baking sheet and set aside. Cut the wonton wrappers in half crosswise, brush them with sesame oil, and arrange them in a single layer on the prepared baking sheet.

2. Sprinkle wonton wrappers with the sesame seeds and salt to taste, and bake until crisp and golden brown, 5 to 7 minutes. Cool completely before serving. These are best eaten on the day they are made but, once cooled, they can be covered and stored at room temperature for 1 to 2 days.

Marinated Mushroom Wraps

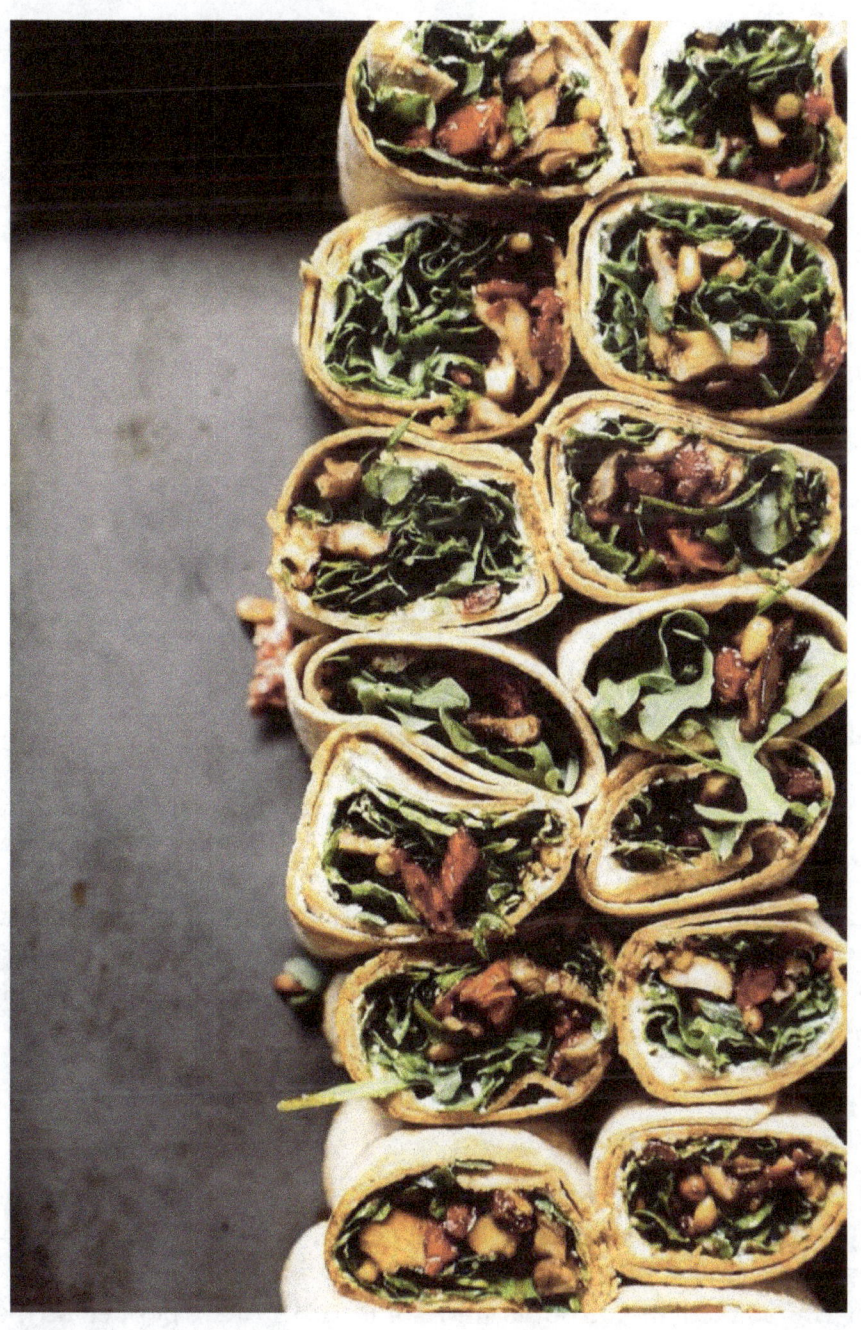

Preparation time: 15 minutes cooking time: 0 minutes servings: 2 wraps

Ingredients

3 tablespoons soy sauce

3 tablespoons fresh lemon juice

1½ tablespoons toasted sesame oil

2 portobello mushroom caps, cut into ¼-inch strips

1 ripe Hass avocado, pitted and peeled

2 (10-inchwhole-grain flour tortillas

2 cups fresh baby spinach leaves

1 medium red bell pepper, cut into ¼-inch strips

1 ripe tomato, chopped

Salt and freshly ground black pepper

Directions

1. In a medium bowl, combine the soy sauce, 2 tablespoons of the lemon juice, and the oil. Add the portobello strips, toss to combine, and marinate for 1 hour or overnight. Drain the mushrooms and set aside.

2. Mash the avocado with the remaining 1 tablespoon of lemon juice.

3. To assemble wraps, place 1 tortilla on a work surface and spread with some of the mashed avocado. Top with a layer of baby spinach leaves. In the lower third of each tortilla, arrange strips of the soaked mushrooms and some of the bell pepper strips.

Sprinkle with the tomato and salt and black pepper to taste. Roll up tightly and cut in half diagonally. Repeat with the remaining Ingredients and serve.

Tamari Toasted Almonds

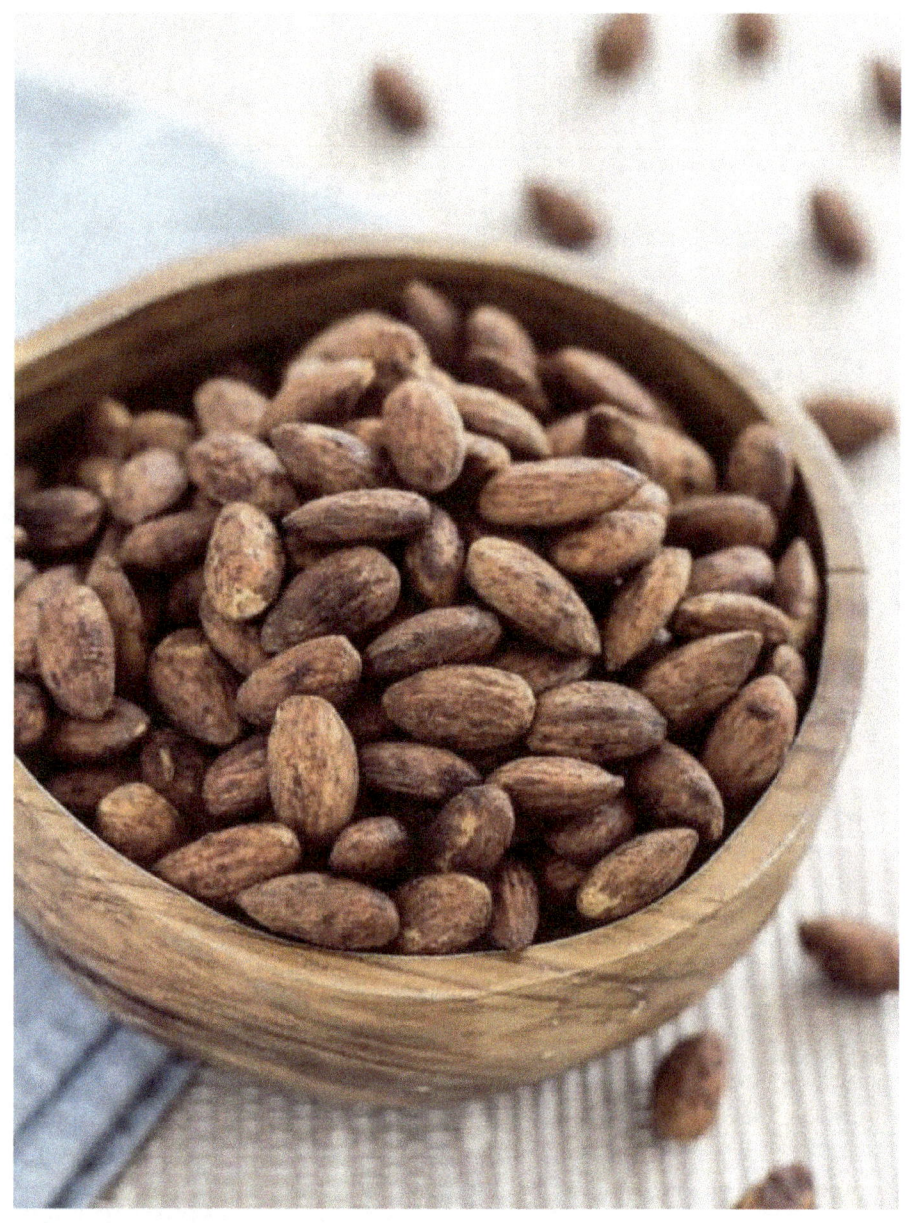

Preparation time: 2 minutes cooking time: 8 minutes servings: ½ cup

Ingredients

½ cup raw almonds, or sunflower seeds

2 tablespoons tamari, or soy sauce

1 teaspoon toasted sesame oil

Directions

1. Heat a dry skillet to medium-high heat, then add the almonds, stirring very frequently to keep them from burning. Once the almonds are toasted, 7 to 8 minutes for almonds, or 3 to 4 minutes for sunflower seeds, pour the tamari and sesame oil into the hot skillet and stir to coat.

2. You can turn off the heat, and as the almonds cool the tamari mixture will stick to and dry on the nuts.

Nutrition (1 tablespoonCalories: 89; Total fat: 8g; Carbs: 3g; Fiber: 2g; Protein: 4g

Avocado And Tempeh Bacon Wraps

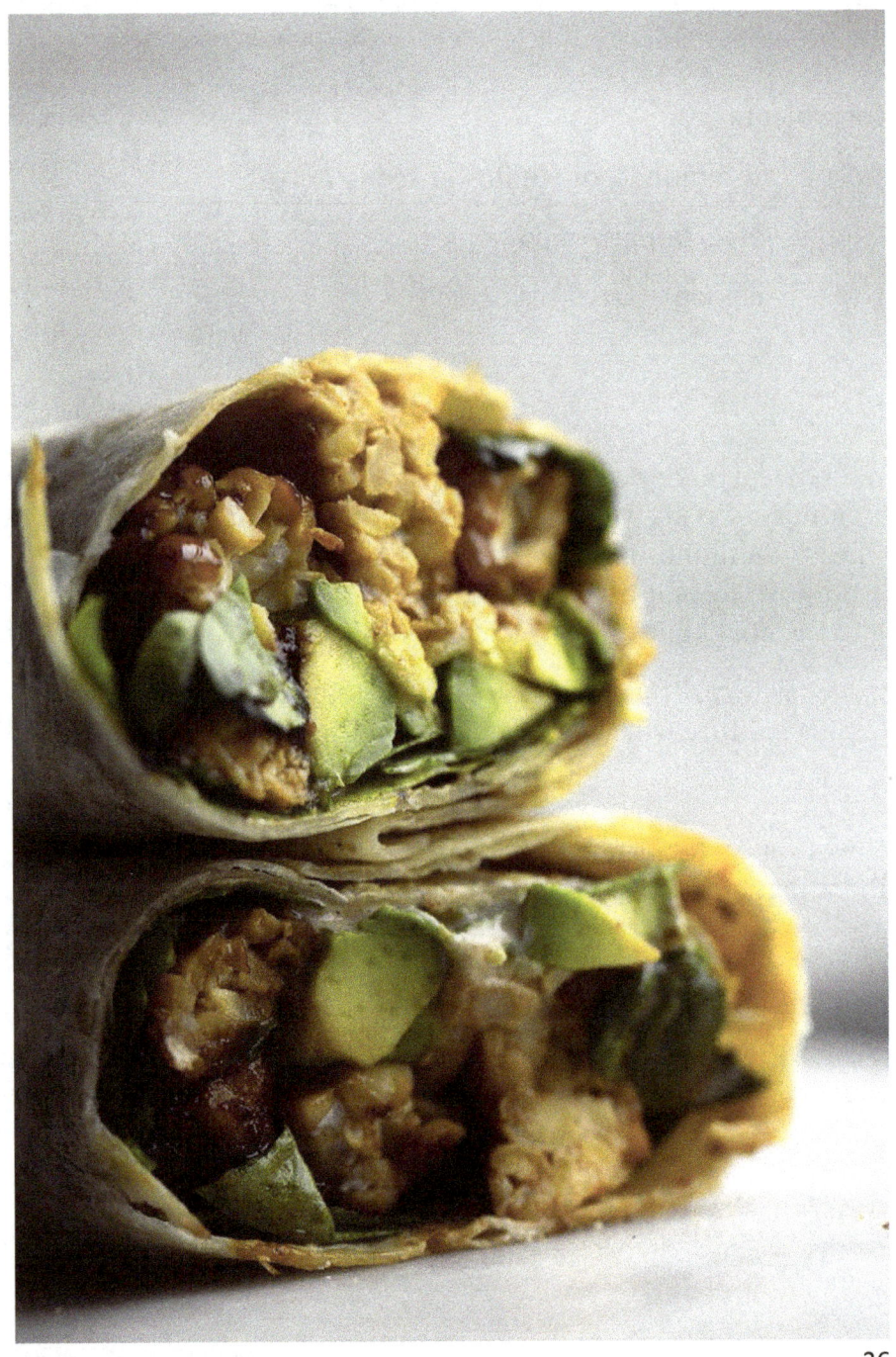

Preparation time: 10 minutes cooking time: 8 minutes servings: 4 wraps

Ingredients

2   tablespoons olive oil

8 ounces tempeh bacon, homemade or store-bought

4 (10-inchsoft flour tortillas or lavash flat bread

¼ cup vegan mayonnaise, homemade or store-bought

4 large lettuce leaves

2 ripe Hass avocados, pitted, peeled, and cut into ¼-inch slices

1 large ripe tomato, cut into ¼-inch slices

Directions

1.   In a large skillet, heat the oil over medium heat. Add the tempeh bacon and cook until browned on both sides, about 8 minutes. Remove from the heat and set aside.

2.   Place 1 tortilla on a work surface. Spread with some of the mayonnaise and one-fourth of the lettuce and tomatoes.

3.   Pit, peel, and thinly slice the avocado and place the slices on top of the tomato. Add the reserved tempeh bacon and roll up tightly. Repeat with remaining Ingredients and serve.

Kale Chips

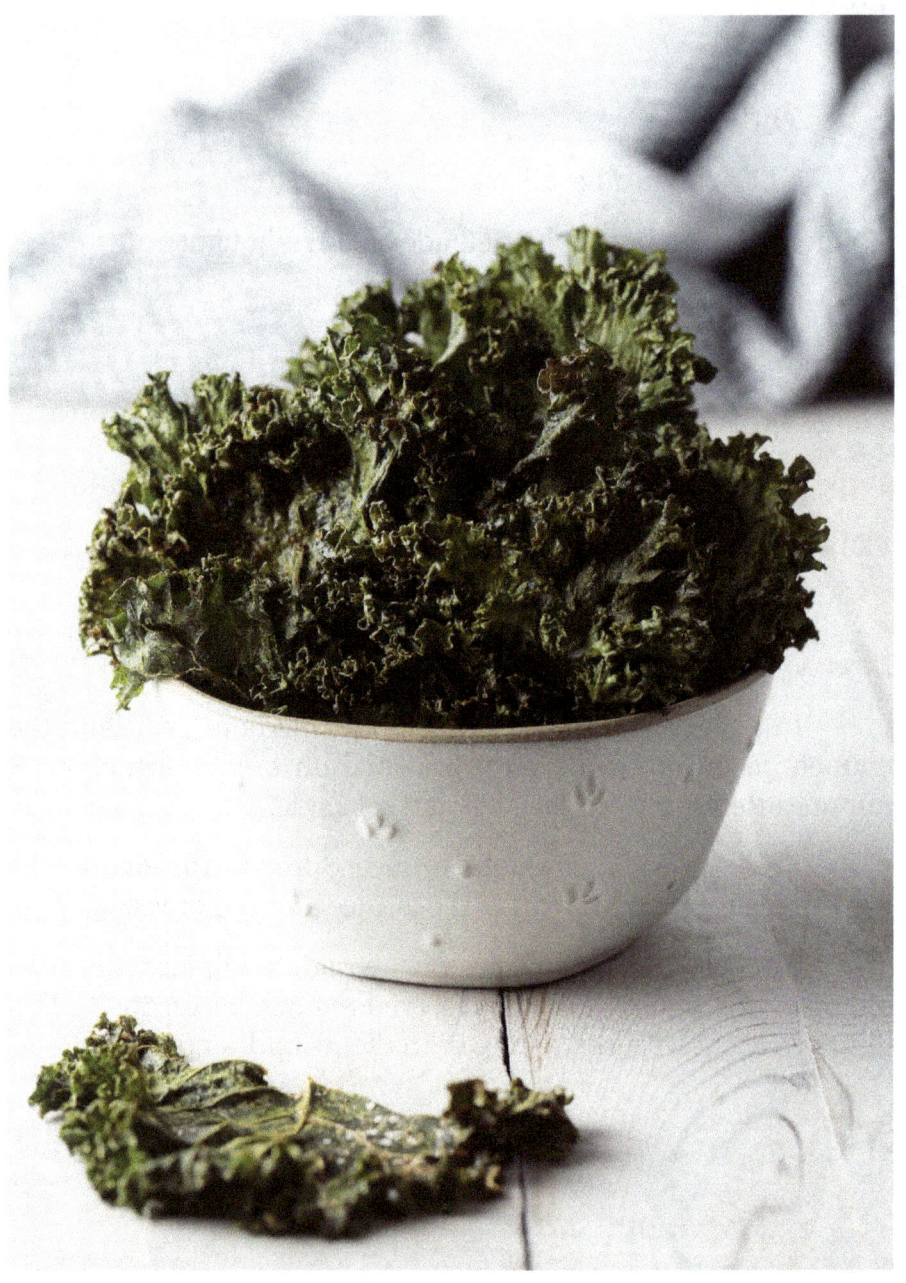

Preparation time: 5 minutes cooking time: 25 minutes servings: 2

Ingredients

1 large bunch kale

1 tablespoon extra-virgin olive oil

½ teaspoon chipotle powder

½ teaspoon smoked paprika

¼ teaspoon salt

Directions

1. Preheat the oven to 275°F.

2. Line a large baking sheet with parchment paper. In a large bowl, stem the kale and tear it into bite-size pieces. Add the olive oil, chipotle powder, smoked paprika, and salt.

3. Toss the kale with tongs or your hands, coating each piece well.

4. Spread the kale over the parchment paper in a single layer.

5. Bake for 25 minutes, turning halfway through, until crisp.

6. Cool for 10 to 15 minutes before dividing and storing in 2 airtight containers.

Nutrition: Calories: 144; Fat: 7g; Protein: 5g; Carbohydrates: 18g; Fiber: 3g; Sugar: 0g; Sodium: 363mg

Tempeh-Pimiento Cheeze Ball

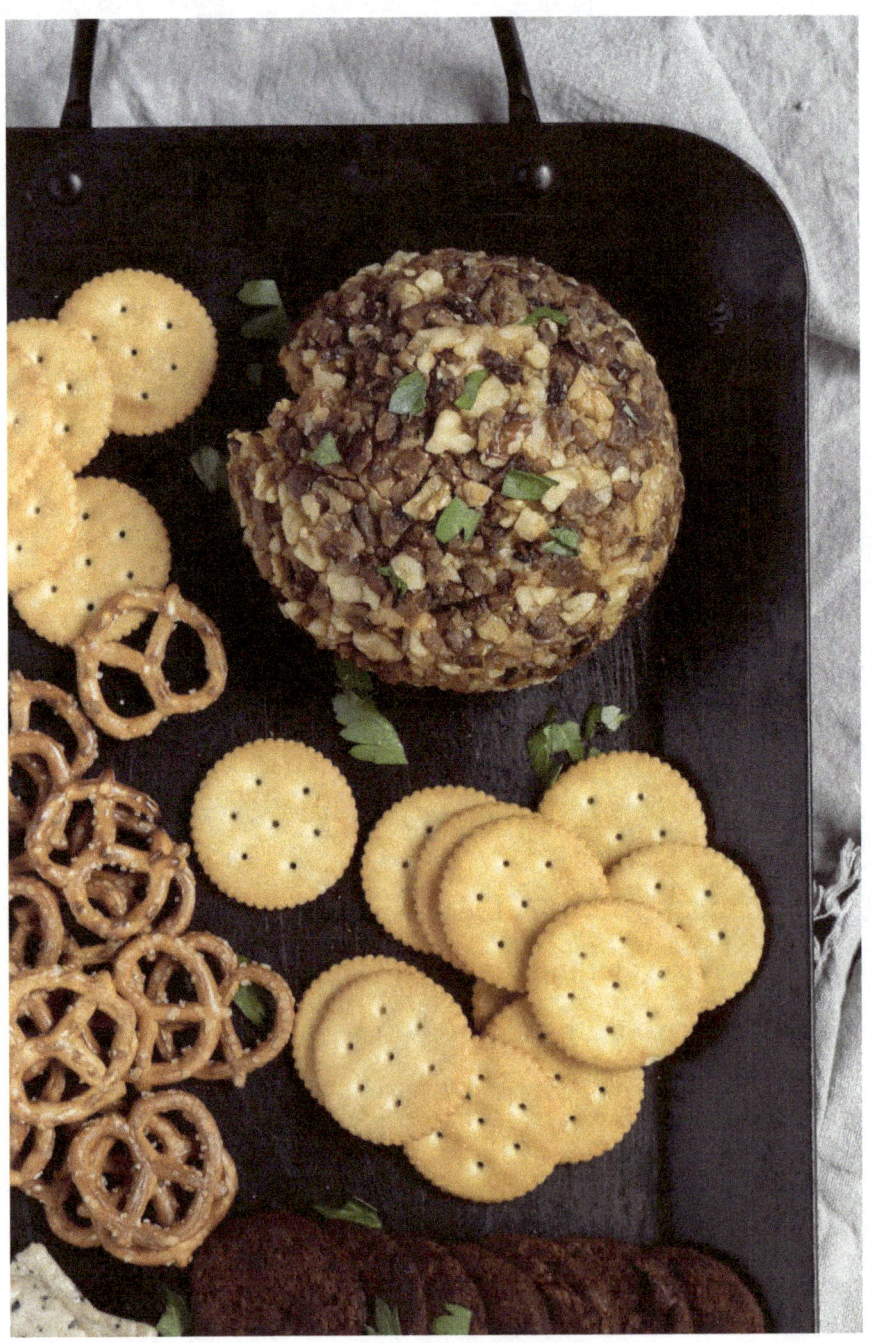

Preparation time: 5 minutes cooking time: 30 minutes servings: 8

Ingredients

8 ounces tempeh, cut into 1/2-inch pieces

1 (2-ouncejar chopped pimientos, drained

1/4 cup nutritional yeast

1/4 cup vegan mayonnaise, homemade or store-bought

2   tablespoons soy sauce

3/4 cup chopped pecans

Directions

1. In a medium saucepan of simmering water, cook the tempeh for 30 minutes. Set aside to cool. In a food processor, combine the cooled tempeh, pimientos, nutritional yeast, mayo, and soy sauce. Process until smooth.

2. Transfer the tempeh mixture to a bowl and refrigerate until firm and chilled, at least 2 hours or overnight.

3. In a dry skillet, toast the pecans over medium heat until lightly toasted, about 5 minutes. Set aside to cool.

4. Shape the tempeh mixture into a ball, and roll it in the pecans, pressing the nuts slightly into the tempeh mixture so they stick. Refrigerate for at least 1 hour before serving. If not using right away, cover and keep refrigerated until needed. Properly stored, it will keep for 2 to 3 days.

Peppers and Hummus

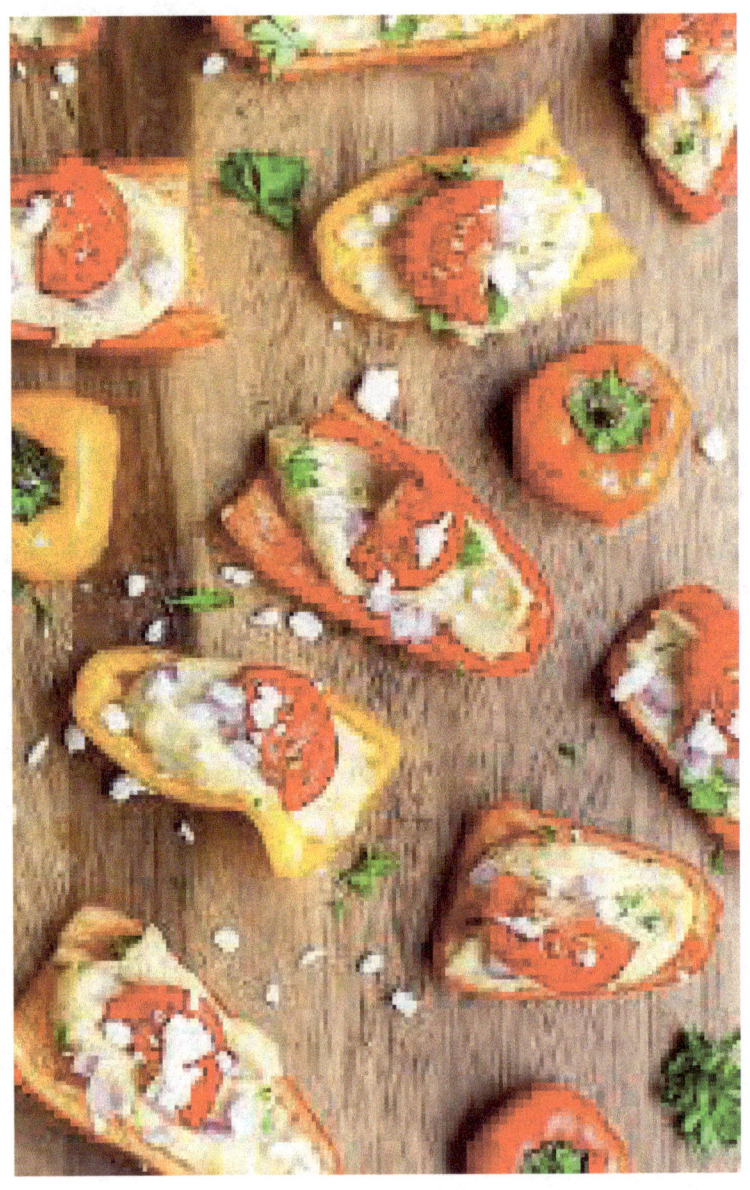

Preparation time: 15 minutes cooking time: 0 minutes servings: 4

Ingredients

one 15-ounce can chickpeas, drained and rinsed

juice of 1 lemon, or 1 tablespoon prepared lemon juice

¼ cup tahini

3   tablespoons olive oil

½ teaspoon ground cumin

1 tablespoon water

¼ teaspoon paprika

1 red bell pepper, sliced

1 green bell pepper, sliced

1 orange bell pepper, sliced

Directions

1.   In a food processor, combine chickpeas, lemon juice, tahini, 2 tablespoons of the olive oil, the cumin, and water.

2.   Process on high speed until blended, about 30 seconds. Scoop the hummus into a bowl and drizzle with the remaining tablespoon of olive oil. Sprinkle with paprika and serve with sliced bell peppers.

Deconstructed Hummus Pitas

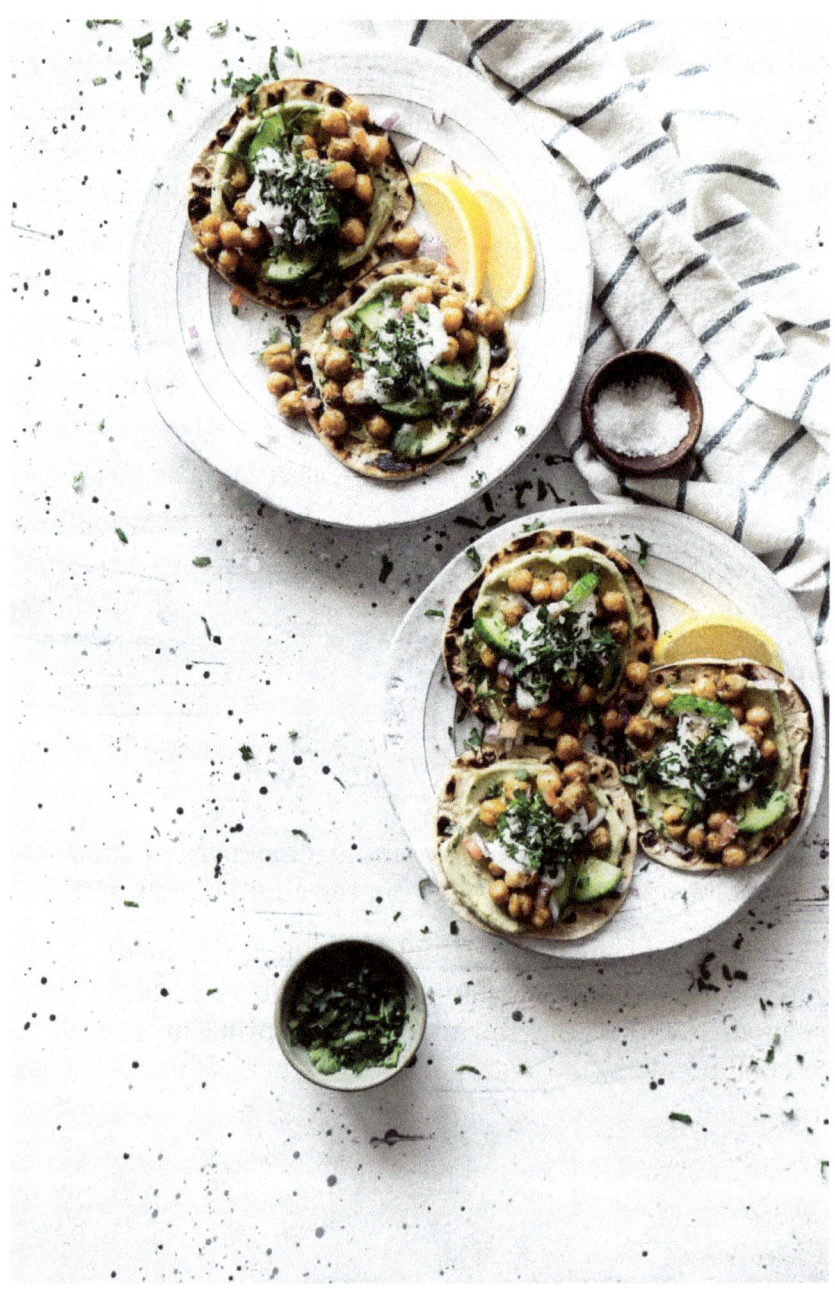

Preparation time: 15 minutes cooking time: 0 minutes servings: 4 pitas

Ingredients

1   garlic clove, crushed

¾ cup tahini (sesame paste

2   tablespoons fresh lemon juice

1 teaspoon salt

⅛ teaspoon ground cayenne

¼ cup water

1½ cups cooked or 1 (15.5-ouncecan chickpeas, rinsed and drained 2 medium carrots, grated (about 1 cup

4 (7-inchpita breads, preferably whole wheat, halved

1 large ripe tomato, cut into ¼-inch slices

2 cups fresh baby spinach

Directions

1. In a blender or food processor, mince the garlic. Add the tahini, lemon juice, salt, cayenne, and water. Process until smooth.

2. Place the chickpeas in a bowl and crush slightly with a fork. Add the carrots and the reserved tahini sauce and toss to combine. Set aside.

3. Spoon 2 or 3 tablespoons of the chickpea mixture into each pita half. Tuck a tomato slice and a few spinach leaves into each pocket and serve.

Savory Roasted Chickpeas

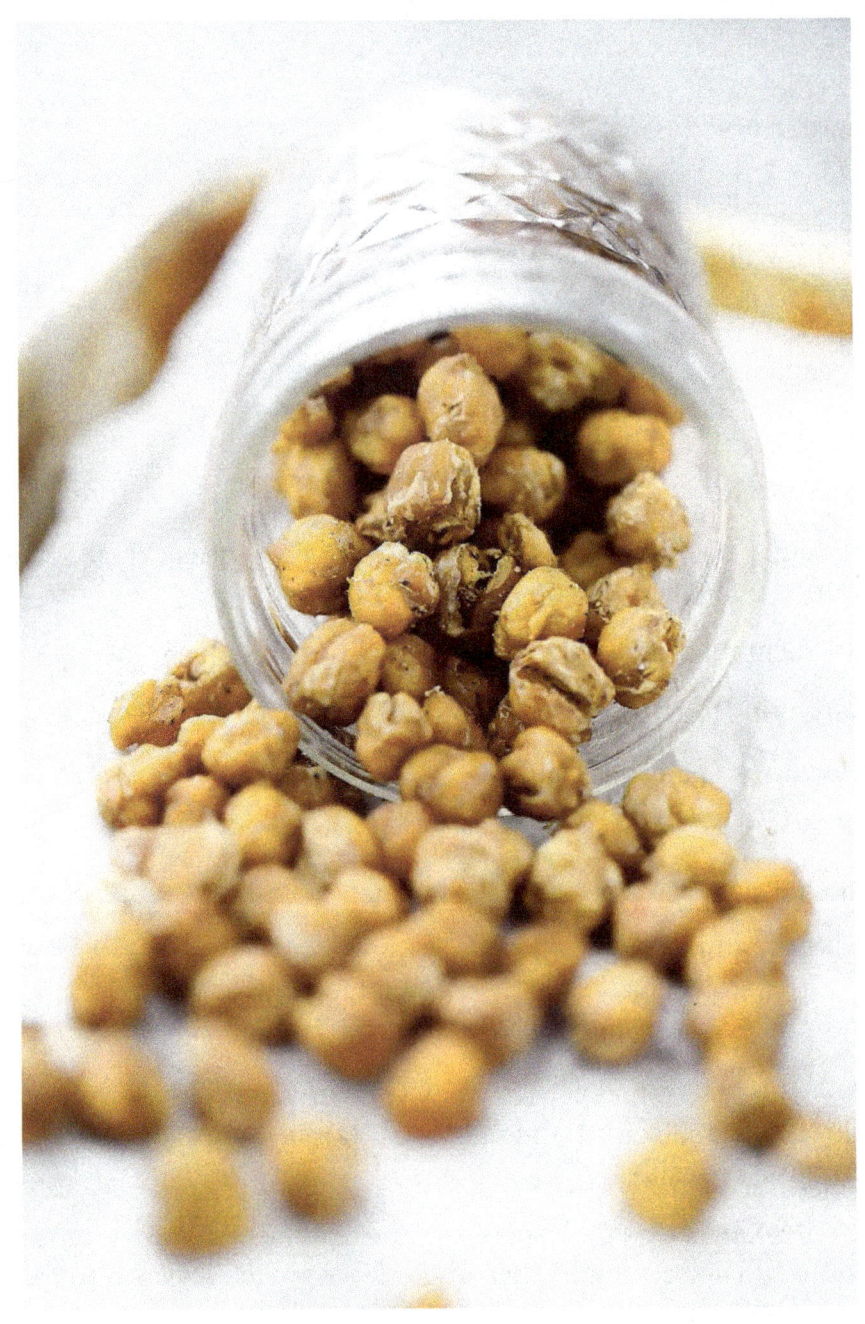

Preparation time: 5 minutes cooking time: 25 minutes servings: 1 cup

Ingredients

1 (14-ouncecan chickpeas, rinsed and drained, or 1½ cups cooked

2 tablespoons tamari, or soy sauce

1 tablespoon nutritional yeast

1 teaspoon smoked paprika, or regular paprika

1 teaspoon onion powder

½ teaspoon garlic powder

Directions

1. Preheat the oven to 400°F.

2. Toss the chickpeas with all the other ingredients, and spread them out on a baking sheet. Bake for 20 to 25 minutes, tossing halfway through.

3. Bake these at a lower temperature, until fully dried and crispy, if you want to keep them longer.

4. You can easily double the batch, and if you dry them out they will keep about a week in an airtight container.

Nutrition (¼ cupCalories: 121; Total fat: 2g; Carbs: 20g; Fiber: 6g; Protein: 8g

Savory Seed Crackers

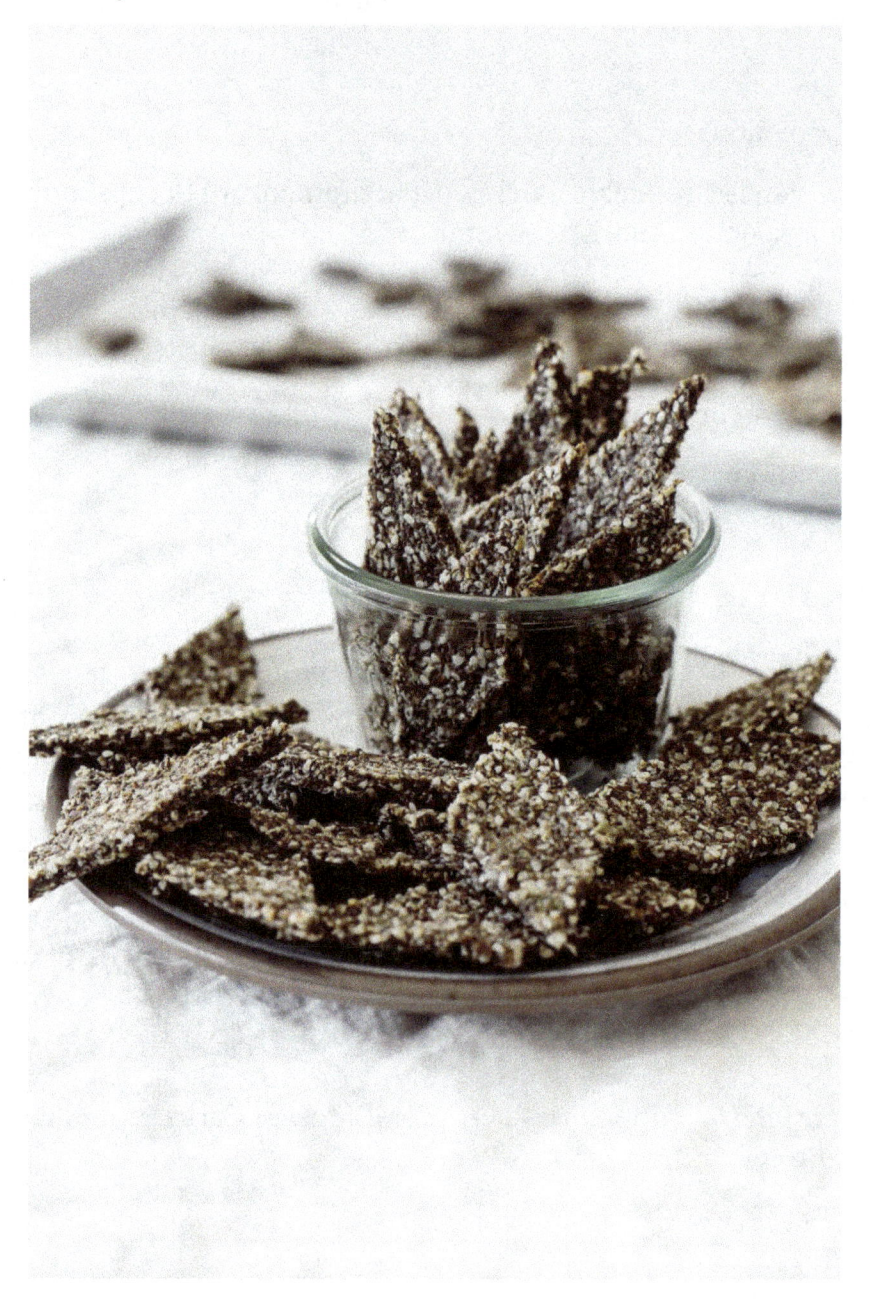

Preparation time: 5 minutes cooking time: 50 minutes servings: 20 crackers

Ingredients

¾ cup pumpkin seeds (pepitas

½ cup sunflower seeds

½ cup sesame seeds

¼ cup chia seeds

1 teaspoon minced garlic (about 1 clove 1 teaspoon tamari or soy sauce

1 teaspoon vegan Worcestershire sauce

½ teaspoon ground cayenne pepper

½ teaspoon dried oregano

½ cup water

Directions

1. Preheat the oven to 325°F.
2. Line a rimmed baking sheet with parchment paper.
3. In a large bowl, combine the pumpkin seeds, sunflower seeds, sesame seeds, chia seeds, garlic, tamari, Worcestershire sauce, cayenne, oregano, and water.
4. Transfer to the prepared baking sheet, spreading out to all sides.

5. Bake for 25 minutes. Remove the pan from the oven, and flip the seed "dough" over so the wet side is up. Bake for another 20 to 25 minutes, until the sides are browned.

6. Cool completely before breaking up into 20 pieces. Divide evenly among 4 glass jars and close tightly with lids.

Nutrition (5 crackers): Calories: 339; Fat: 29g; Protein: 14g; Carbohydrates: 17g; Fiber: 8g; Sugar: 1g; Sodium: 96mg

Tomato and Basil Bruschetta

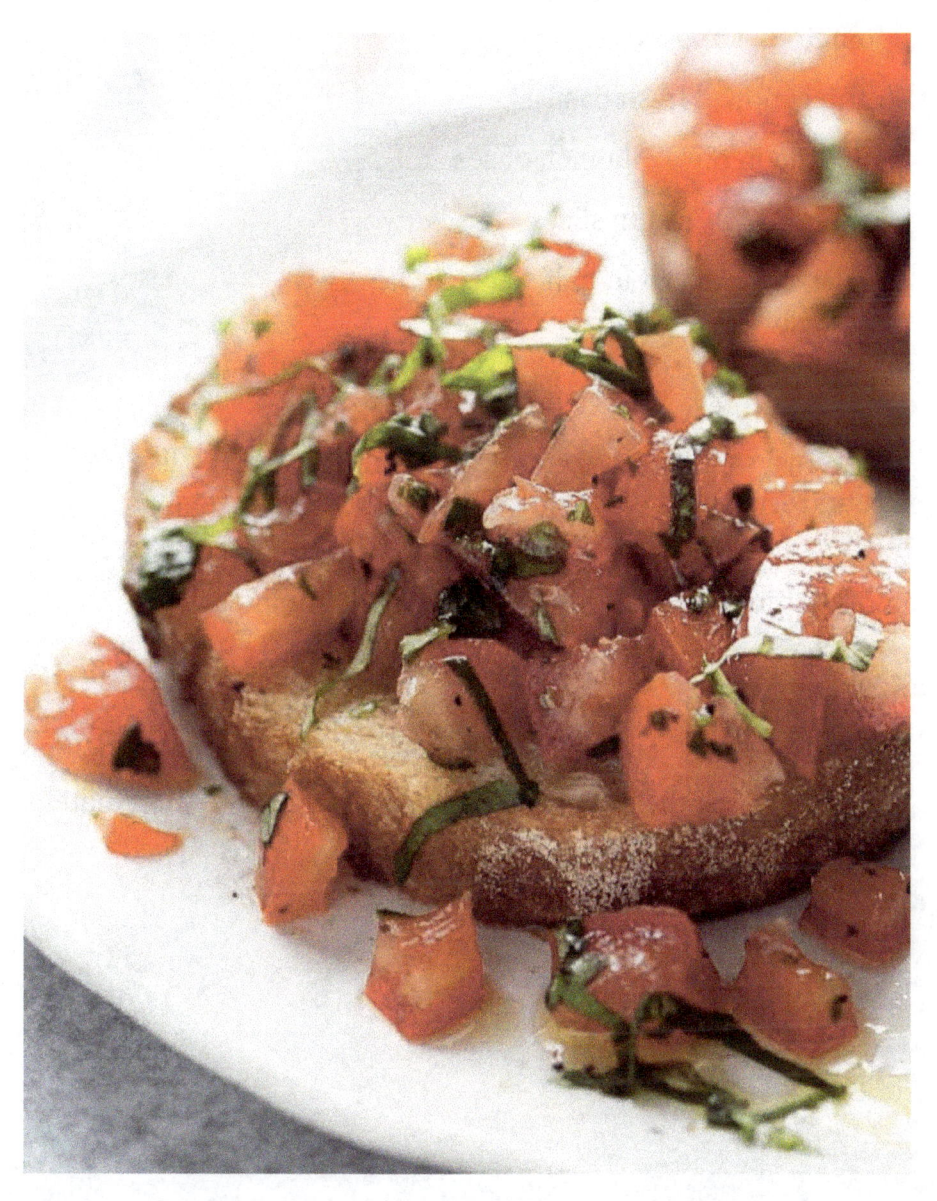

Preparation time: 10 minutes cooking time: 6 minutes servings: 12 bruschetta

Ingredients

3 tomatoes, chopped

¼ cup chopped fresh basil

1 tablespoon olive oil pinch of sea salt

1 baguette, cut into 12 slices

1 garlic clove, sliced in half

Directions

1. In a small bowl, combine the tomatoes, basil, olive oil, and salt and stir to mix. Set aside. Preheat the oven to 425°F.

2. Place the baguette slices in a single layer on a baking sheet and toast in the oven until brown, about 6 minutes.

3. Flip the bread slices over once during cooking. Remove from the oven and rub the bread on both sides with the sliced clove of garlic.

4. Top with the tomato-basil mixture and serve immediately.

Refried Bean And Salsa Quesadillas

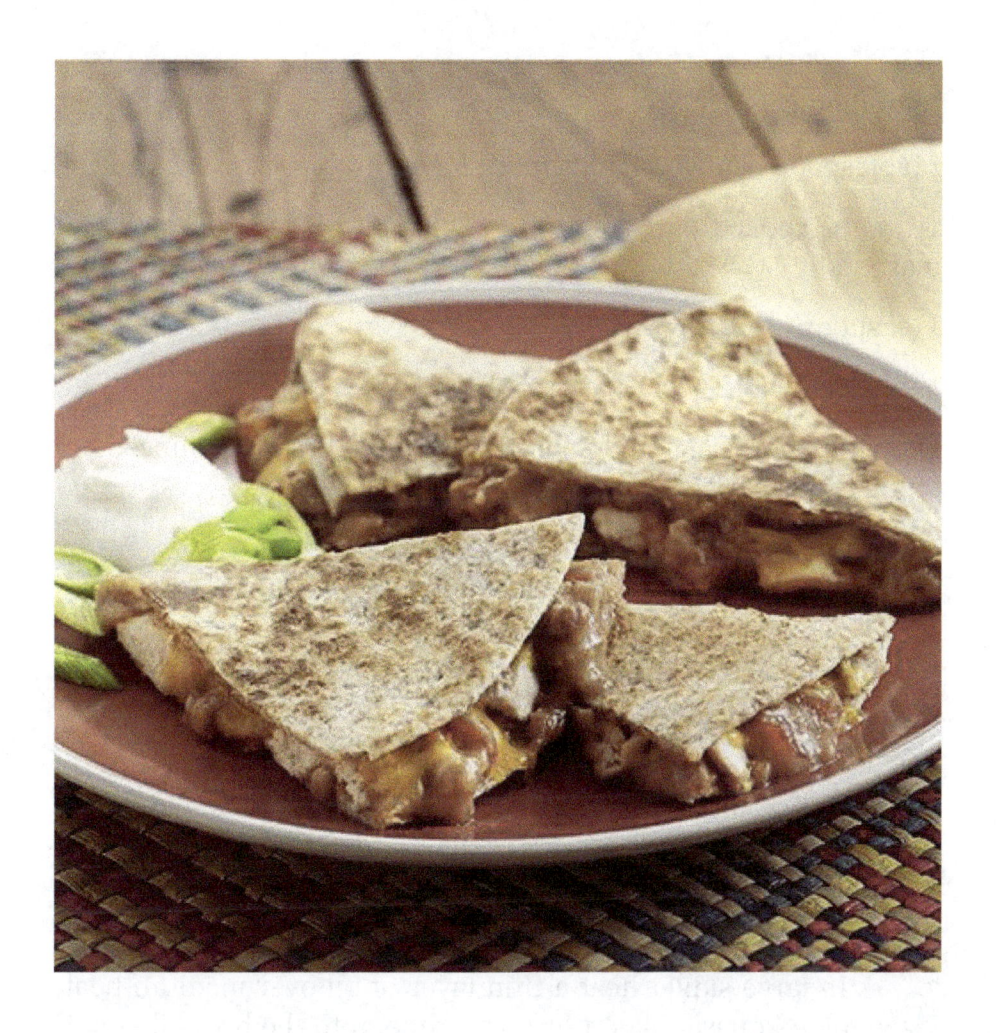

Preparation time: 5 minutes cooking time: 6 minutes servings: 4 quesadillas

Ingredients

1 tablespoon canola oil, plus more for frying

1½ cups cooked or 1 (15.5-ouncecan pinto beans, drained and mashed

1 teaspoon chili powder

4 (10-inchwhole-wheat flour tortillas

1 cup tomato salsa, homemade or store-bought ½ cup minced red onion (optional

Directions

1. In a medium saucepan, heat the oil over medium heat. Add the mashed beans and chili powder and cook, stirring, until hot, about 5 minutes. Set aside.

2. To assemble, place 1 tortilla on a work surface and spoon about ¼ cup of the beans across the bottom half. Top the beans with the salsa and onion, if using. Fold top half of the tortilla over the filling and press slightly.

3. In large skillet heat a thin layer of oil over medium heat. Place folded quesadillas, 1 or 2 at a time, into the hot skillet and heat until hot, turning once, about 1 minute per side.

4. Cut quesadillas into 3 or 4 wedges and arrange on plates. Serve immediately.

Tempeh Tantrum Burgers

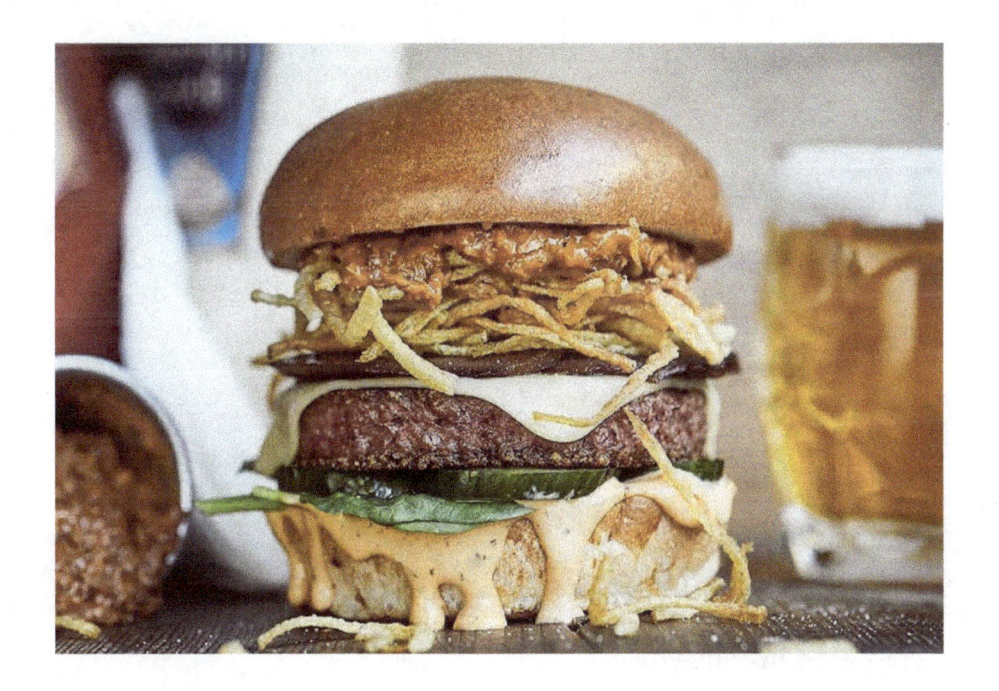

Preparation time: 15 minutes

cooking time: 0 minutes servings: 4 burgers

Ingredients

8 ounces tempeh, cut into 1/2-inch dice

3/4 cup chopped onion

2 garlic cloves, chopped

3/4 cup chopped walnuts

1/2 cup old-fashioned or quick-cooking oats

1 tablespoon minced fresh parsley

1/2 teaspoon dried oregano

1/2 teaspoon dried thyme

1/2 teaspoon salt

1/4 teaspoon freshly ground black pepper

3 tablespoons olive oil

Dijon mustard

4 whole grain burger rolls

Sliced red onion, tomato, lettuce, and avocado

Directions

1. In a medium saucepan of simmering water, cook the tempeh for 30 minutes. Drain and set aside to cool.

2. In a food processor, combine the onion and garlic and process until minced. Add the cooled tempeh, the walnuts, oats, parsley, oregano, thyme, salt, and pepper. Process until well blended. Shape the mixture into 4 equal patties.

3. In a large skillet, heat the oil over medium heat. Add the burgers and cook until cooked thoroughly and browned on both sides, about 7 minutes per side.

4. Spread desired amount of mustard onto each half of the rolls and layer each roll with lettuce, tomato, red onion, and avocado, as desired. Serve immediately.

Sesame- Wonton Crisps

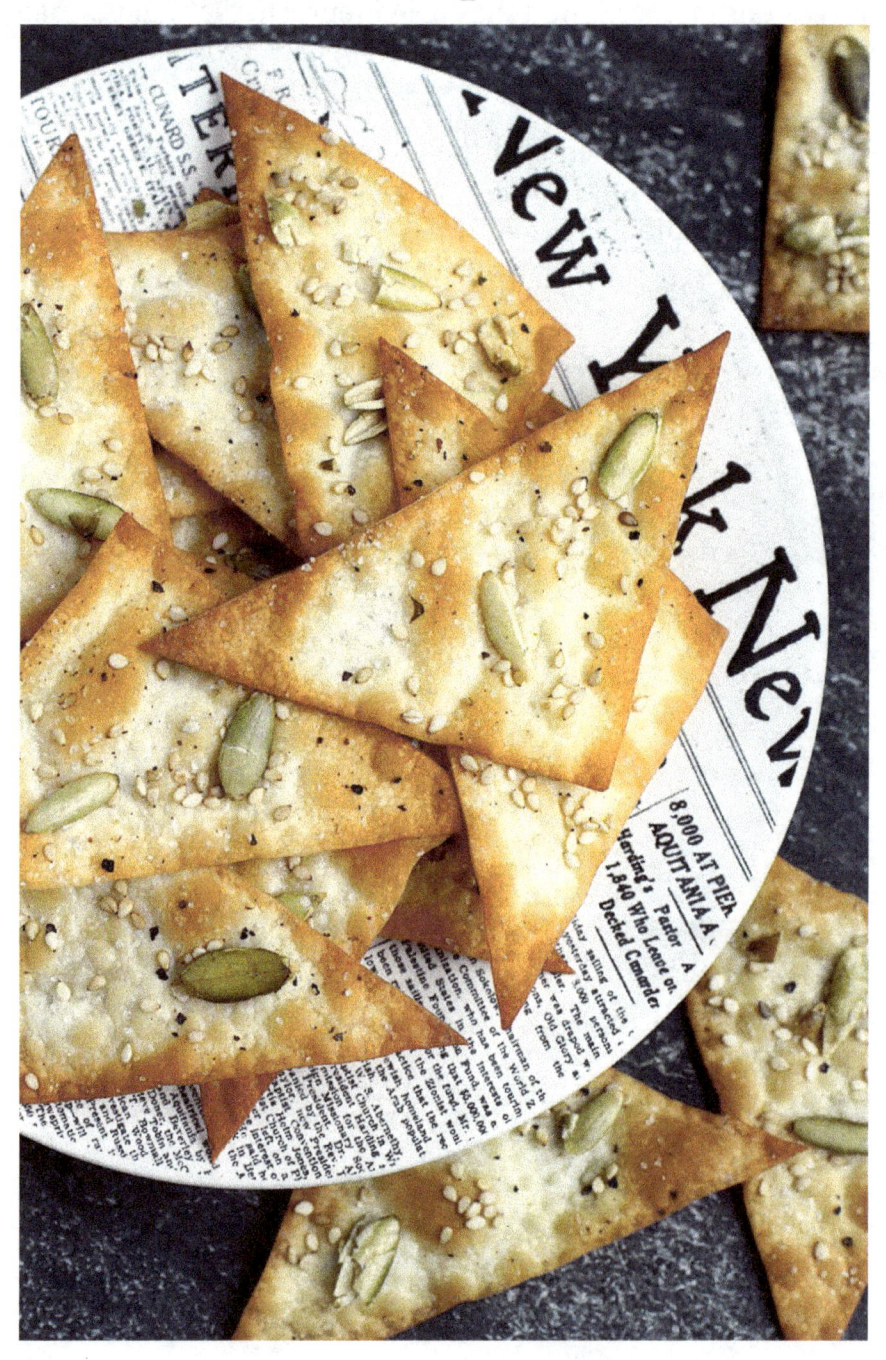

Preparation time: 10 minutes cooking time: 10 minutes

servings: 12 crisps

Ingredients

12 Vegan Wonton Wrappers

2 tablespoons toasted sesame oil

12 shiitake mushrooms, lightly rinsed, patted dry, stemmed, and cut into 1/4-inch slices

4 snow peas, trimmed and cut crosswise into thin slivers

1 teaspoon soy sauce

1 tablespoon fresh lime juice

1/2 teaspoon brown sugar

1 medium carrot, shredded

Toasted sesame seeds or black sesame seeds, if available

Directions

1.   Preheat the oven to 350°F. Lightly oil a baking sheet and set aside. Brush the wonton wrappers with 1 tablespoon of the sesame oil and arrange on the baking sheet. Bake until golden brown and crisp, about 5 minutes. Set aside to cool. (Alternately, you can tuck the wonton wrappers into mini-muffin tins to create cups for the filling. Brush with sesame oil and bake them until crisp.

2.   In a large skillet, heat the extra olive oil over medium heat. Add the mushrooms and cook until softened, 3 to 5 minutes. Stir in the snow peas and the soy sauce and cook 30 seconds. Set aside to cool.

3. In a large bowl, combine the lime juice, sugar, and remaining 1 tablespoon sesame oil. Stir in the carrot and cooled shiitake mixture. Top each wonton crisp with a spoonful of the shiitake mixture. Sprinkle with sesame seeds and arrange on a platter to serve.

Macadamia-Cashew Patties

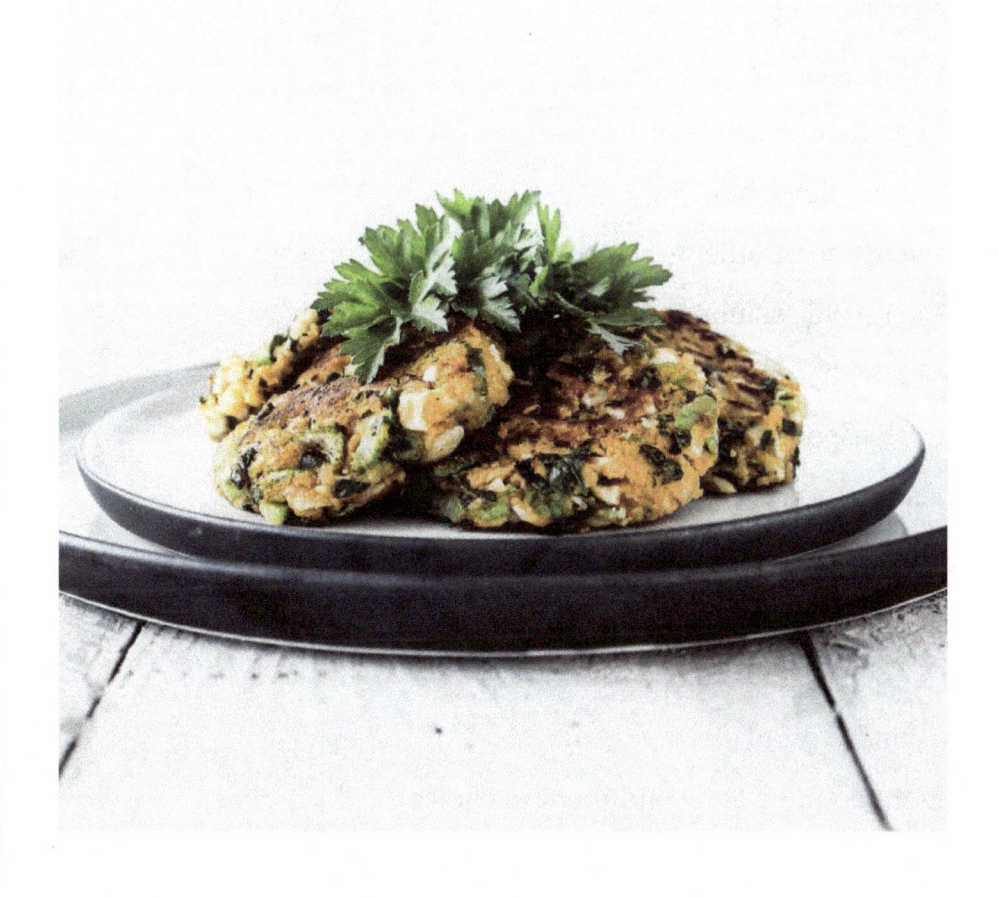

Preparation time: 10 minutes cooking time: 10 minutes servings: 4 patties

Ingredients

¾ cup chopped macadamia nuts

¾ cup chopped cashews

1 medium carrot, grated

1 small onion, chopped

1 garlic clove, minced

1 jalapeño or other green chile, seeded and minced

¾ cup old-fashioned oats

¾ cup dry unseasoned bread crumbs

2 tablespoons minced fresh cilantro

½ teaspoon ground coriander

Salt and freshly ground black pepper

2 teaspoons fresh lime juice

Canola or grapeseed oil, for frying

4 sandwich rolls

Lettuce leaves and condiment of choice

Directions

1. In a food processor, combine the macadamia nuts, cashews, carrot, onion, garlic, chile, oats, bread crumbs, cilantro, coriander, and salt and pepper to taste. Process until well mixed. Add the lime juice and process until well blended. Taste,

adjusting seasonings if necessary. Shape the mixture into 4 equal patties.

2. In a large skillet, heat a thin layer of oil over medium heat. Add the patties and cook until golden brown on both sides, turning once, about 10 minutes total. Serve on sandwich rolls with lettuce and condiments of choice.

Garlic Tahini Spread

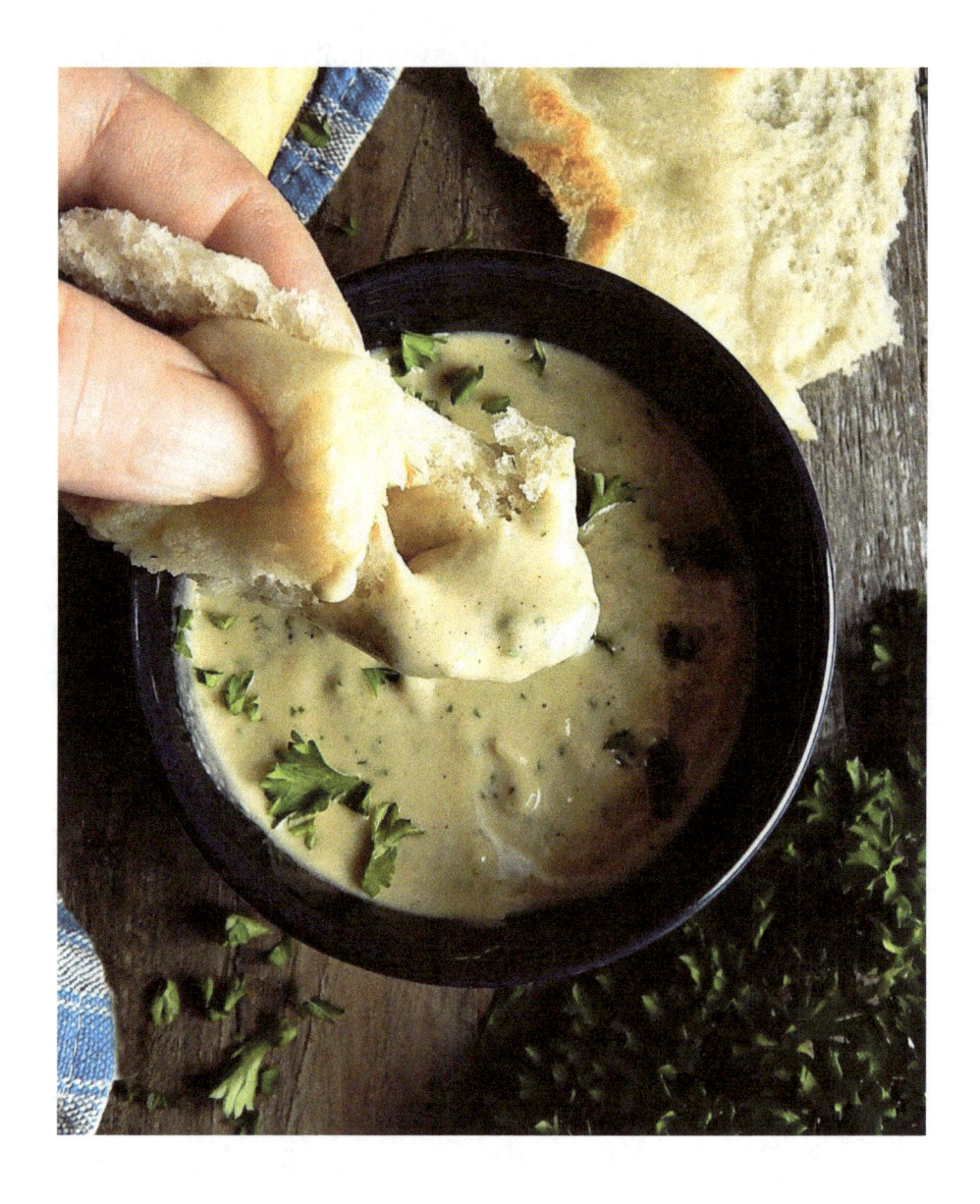

Preparation time: 10 minutes Cooking time: 15 minutes Servings: 4

Ingredients:

1   cup coconut cream

2   tablespoons tahini paste

4 garlic cloves, minced

Juice of 1 lime

¼ teaspoon turmeric powder

A pinch of salt and black pepper

1 teaspoon sweet paprika

1 tablespoon olive oil

Directions:

1.   Heat up a pan with the oil over medium heat, add the garlic, turmeric and paprika and cook for 5 minutes.

2.   Add the rest of the ingredients, stir, cook over medium heat for 10 minutes more, blend using an immersion blender, divide into bowls and serve.

Nutrition: calories 170, fat 7.3, fiber 4, carbs 1, protein 5

Balsamic Pearl Onions Bowls

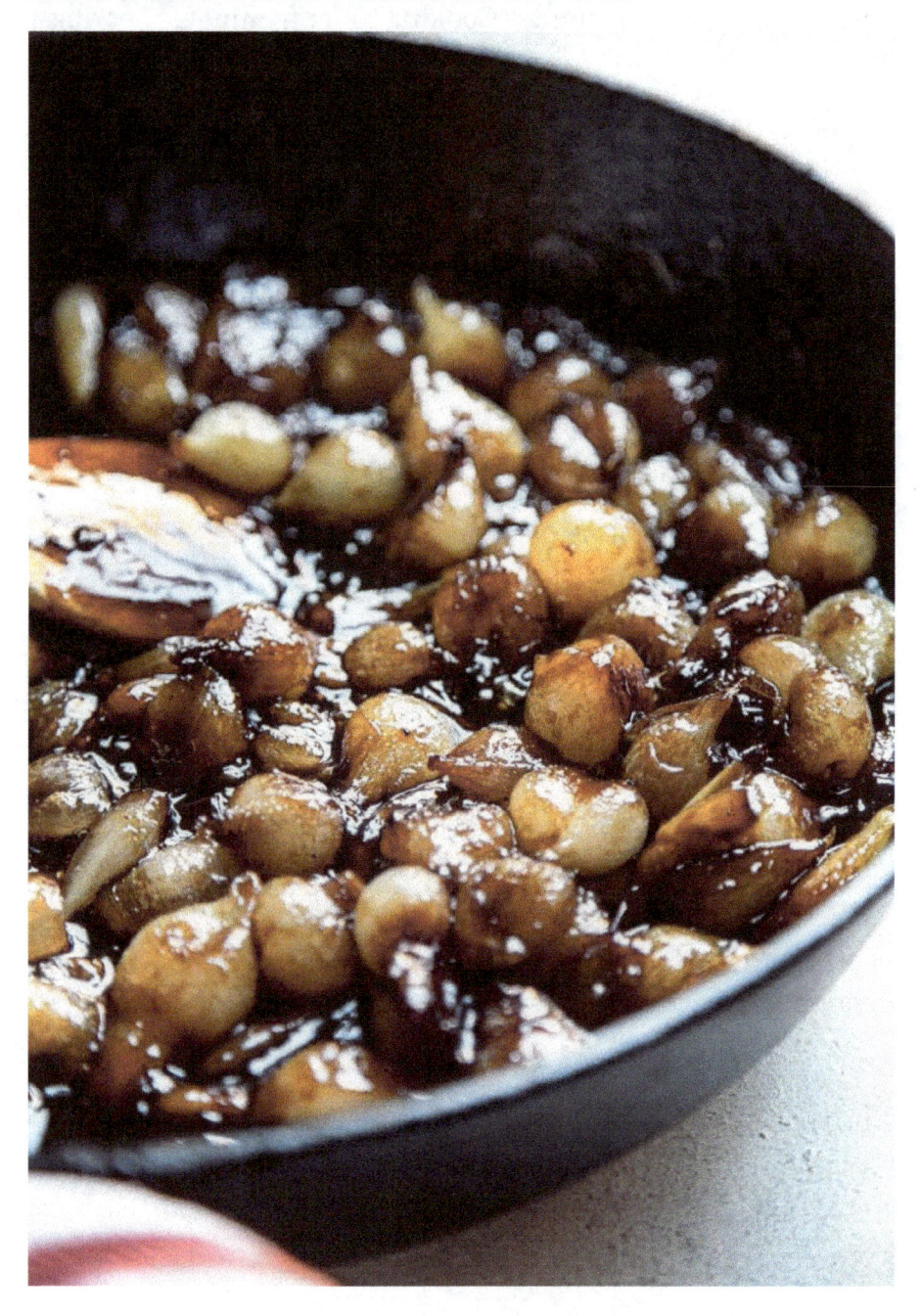

Preparation time: 5 minutes Cooking time: 15 minutes Servings: 4

Ingredients:

1 pound pearl onions, peeled

A pinch of salt and black pepper

2 tablespoons avocado oil

4 tablespoons balsamic vinegar

1 tablespoon chives, chopped

Directions:

1. Heat up a pan with the oil over medium heat, add the pearl onions, salt, pepper and the other ingredients, cook for 15 minutes, divide into bowls and serve as a snack.

Nutrition: calories 120, fat 2, fiber 1, carbs 2, protein 2

Basil Rice Bowls

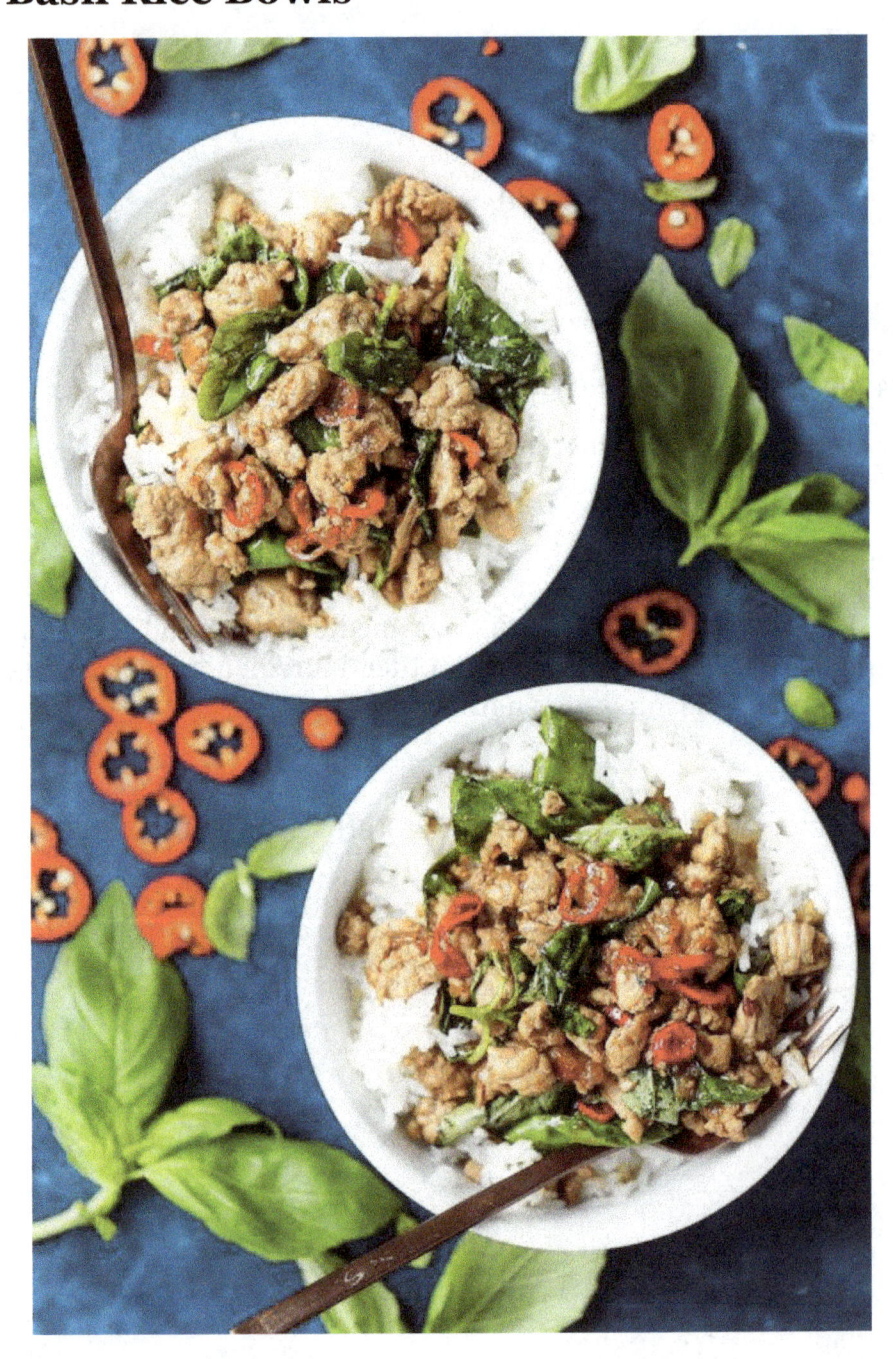

Preparation time: 10 minutes Cooking time: 20 minutes Servings: 4

Ingredients:

2 cups cauliflower rice

1 cup veggie stock

A pinch of salt and black pepper

1 teaspoon turmeric powder

1 teaspoon cumin, ground

1 teaspoon fennel seeds, crushed

2 tablespoons olive oil

2 tomatoes, cubed

1 cup black olives, pitted and sliced

1 bunch basil, chopped

Directions:

1. Heat up a pan with the oil over medium heat, add the cauliflower rice, stock, salt, pepper and the other ingredients, stir, cook for 20 minutes, divide into small bowls and serve as an appetizer.

Nutrition: calories 118, fat 11.5, fiber 2.2, carbs 5.9, protein 4

Turmeric Peppers Platter

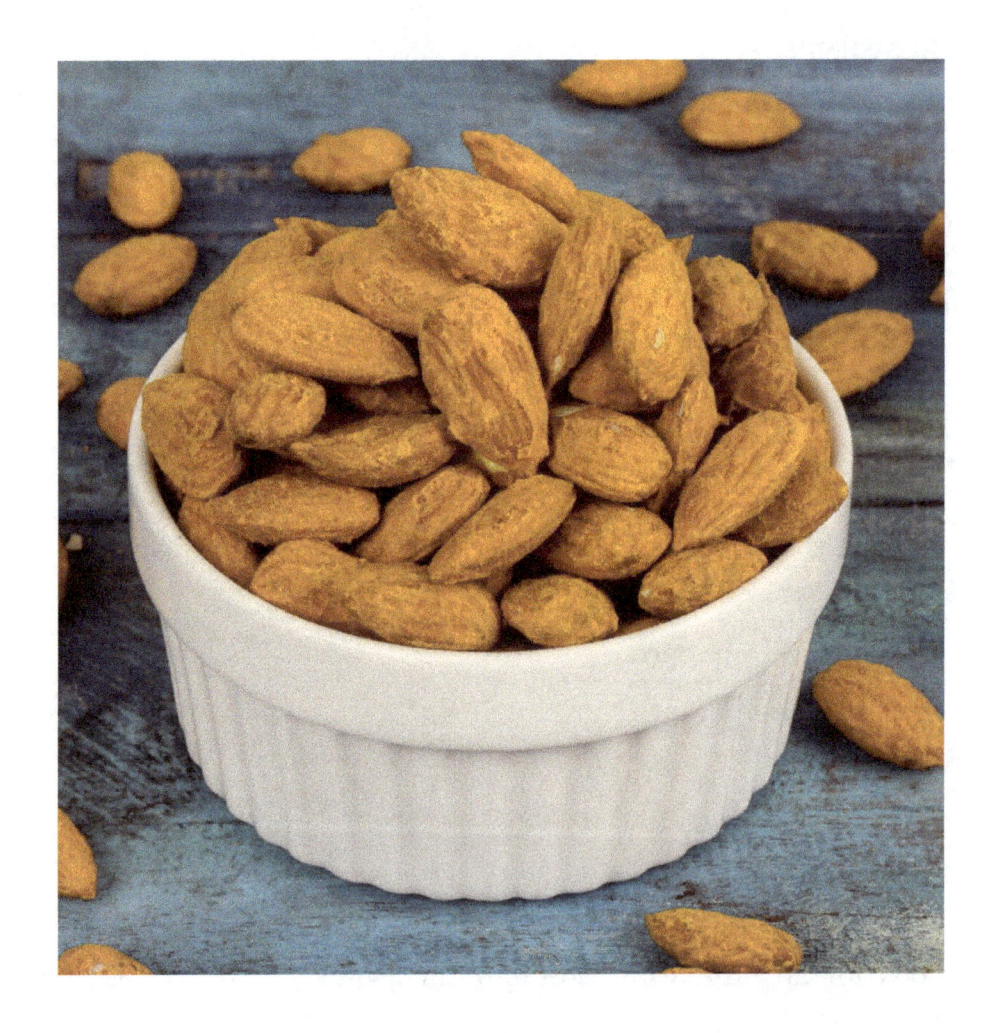

Preparation time: 10 minutes Cooking time: 20 minutes

Servings: 4

Ingredients:

2   green bell peppers, cut into wedges

2 red bell peppers, cut into wedges

2 yellow bell peppers, cut into wedges

2 tablespoons avocado oil

2 garlic cloves, minced

1 bunch basil, chopped

A pinch of salt and black pepper

2 tablespoons balsamic vinegar

Directions:

1.   Heat up a pan with the oil over medium heat, add the garlic and the vinegar and cook for 2 minutes.

2.   Add the peppers and the other ingredients, toss, cook over medium heat for 18 minutes, arrange them on a platter and serve as an appetizer.

Nutrition: calories 120, fat 8.2, fiber 2, carbs 4, protein 2.3

Capers Dip

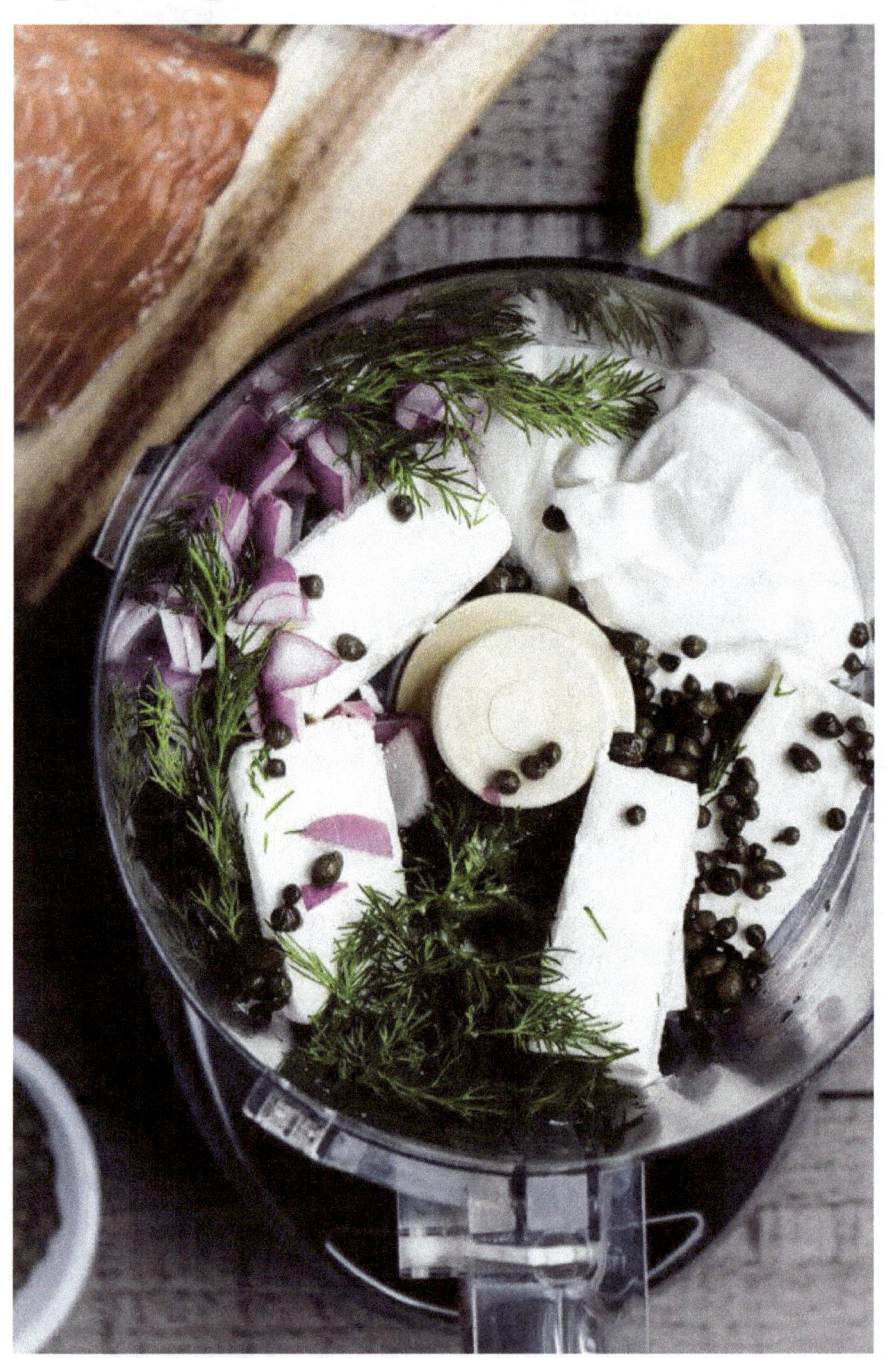

Preparation time: 10 minutes Cooking time: 20 minutes Servings: 4

Ingredients:

2 tablespoons olive oil

4 scallions, chopped

1 teaspoon rosemary, dried

2 tablespoons capers, drained

1 cup coconut cream

2 tablespoons pine nuts

1 bunch basil, chopped

Directions:

1. Heat up a pan with the oil over medium heat, add the scallions and the capers and sauté for 5 minutes.

2. Add the cream and the other ingredients, stir, cook over medium heat for 15 minutes more, blend using an immersion blender, divide into bowls and serve.

Nutrition: calories 127, fat 3, fiber 3, carbs 6, protein 7

Radish and Walnuts Dip

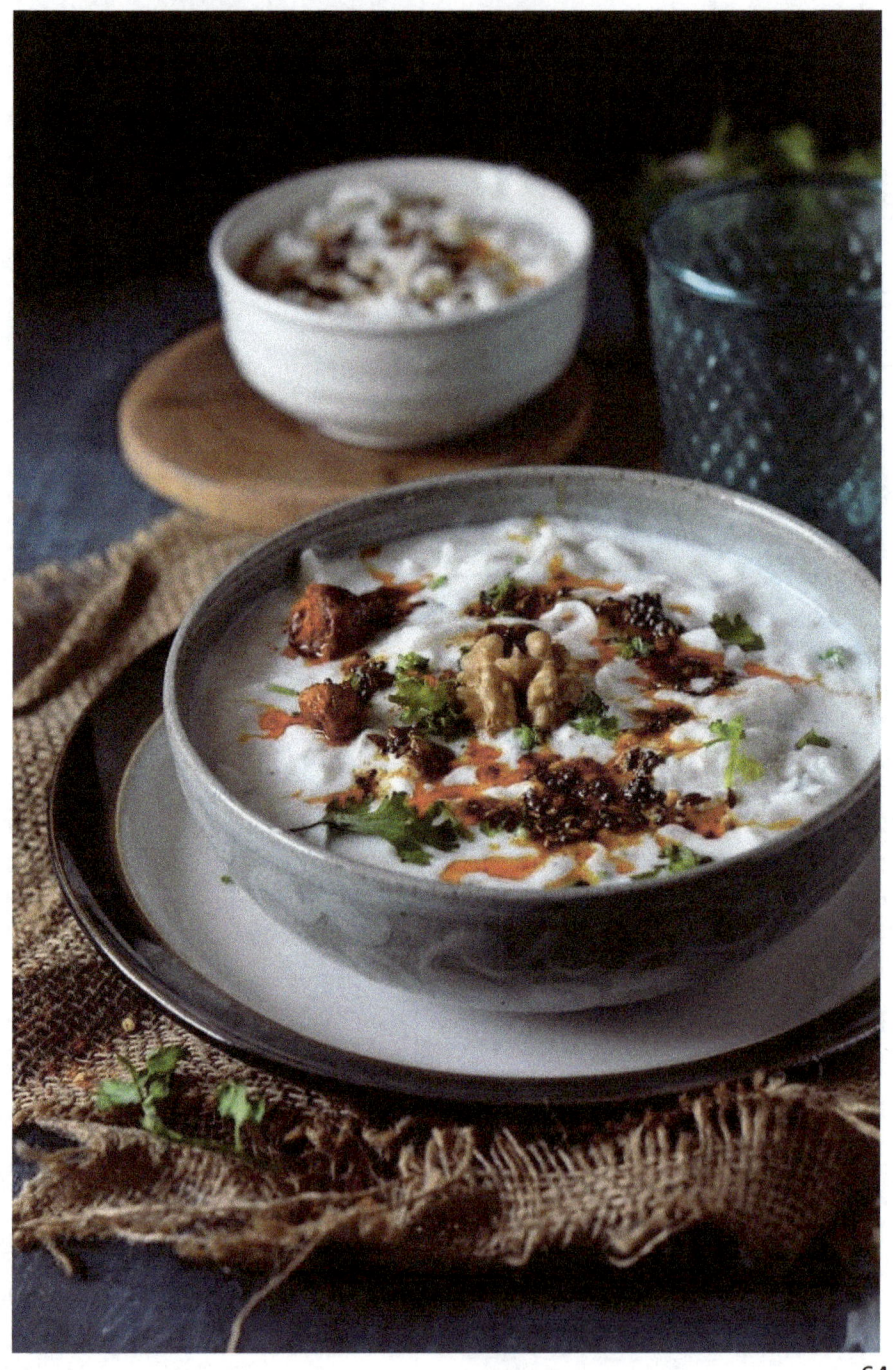

Preparation time: 10 minutes Cooking time: 20 minutes

Servings: 4

Ingredients:

2 tablespoons walnuts, chopped

1 cup coconut cream

2 cups radishes, chopped

4 scallions, chopped

2 tablespoons olive oil

1 teaspoon chili powder

A pinch of salt and black pepper

2 teaspoons mustard powder

2 teaspoons garlic powder

2 teaspoons cumin, ground

Directions:

1. Heat up a pan with the oil over medium heat, add the scallions, mustard powder, garlic powder and cumin, stir and sauté for 5 minutes.

2. Add the walnuts, and the other ingredients, stir, cook over medium heat for 15 minutes, blend well using an immersion blender, divide into bowls and serve.

Nutrition: calories 192, fat 5, fiber 7, carbs 12, protein 5

Mushroom Cakes

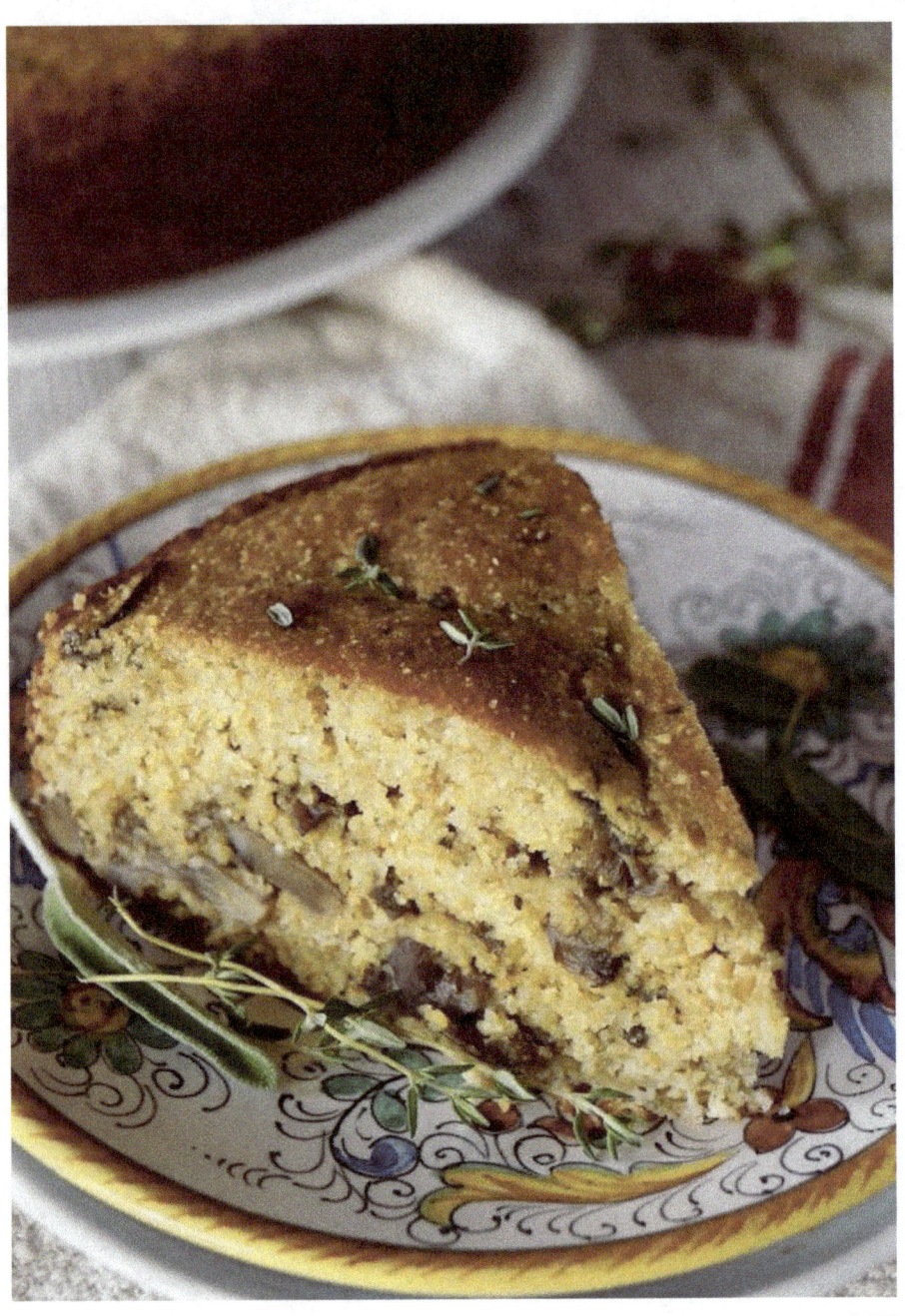

Preparation time: 10 minutes

Cooking time: 12 minutes Servings: 6

Ingredients:

1 cup shallots, chopped

2 tablespoons olive oil

3 garlic cloves, minced

1 pound mushrooms, minced

2 tablespoons almond flour

¼ cup coconut cream

1 tablespoon flaxseed mixed with

2 tablespoons water

¼ cup parsley, chopped

Directions:

1. In a bowl, combine the shallots with the garlic, the mushrooms and the other ingredients except the oil, stir well and shape medium cakes out of this mix.

2. Heat up a pan with the oil over medium heat, add the mushroom cakes, cook for 6 minutes on each side, arrange them on a platter and serve as an appetizer.

Nutrition: calories 222, fat 4, fiber 3, carbs 8, protein 10

Cabbage Sticks

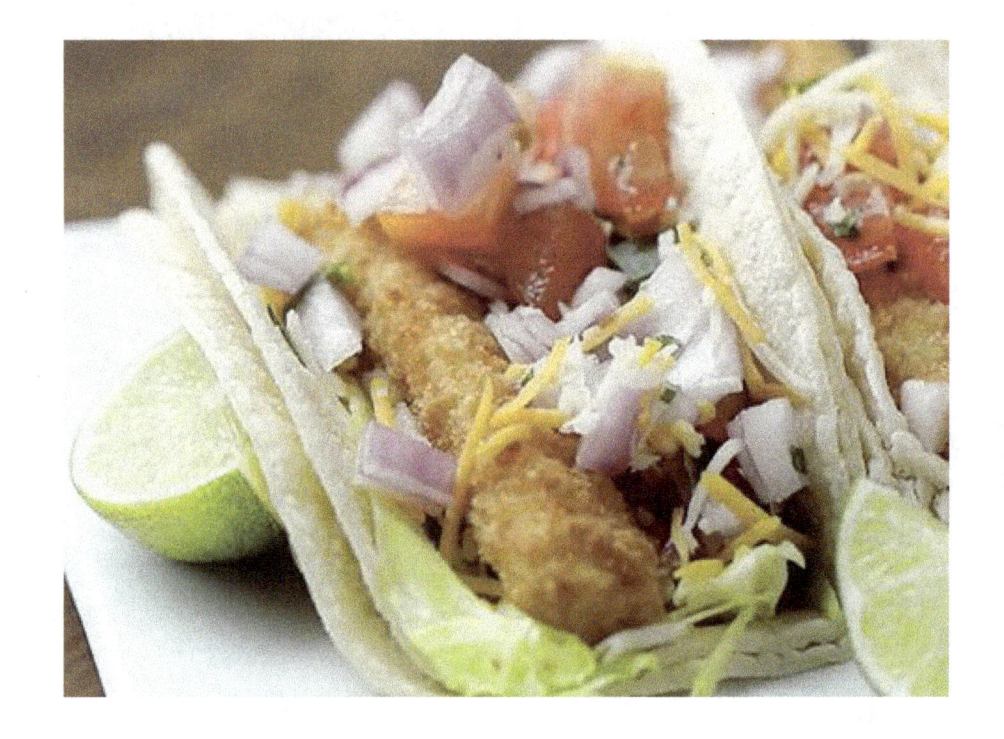

Preparation time: 10 minutes Cooking time: 30 minutes Servings: 4

Ingredients:

1 pound cabbage, leaves separated and cut into thick strips

1 tablespoon olive oil

1 tablespoon balsamic vinegar

1 teaspoon ginger, grated

1 teaspoon hot paprika

A pinch of salt and black pepper

Directions:

1. Spread the cabbage strips on a baking sheet lined with parchment paper, add the oil, the vinegar and the other ingredients, toss and cook at 400 degrees F for 30 minutes.

2. Divide the cabbage strips into bowls and serve as a snack.

Nutrition: calories 300, fat 4, fiber 7, carbs 18, protein 6

Crispy Brussels Sprouts

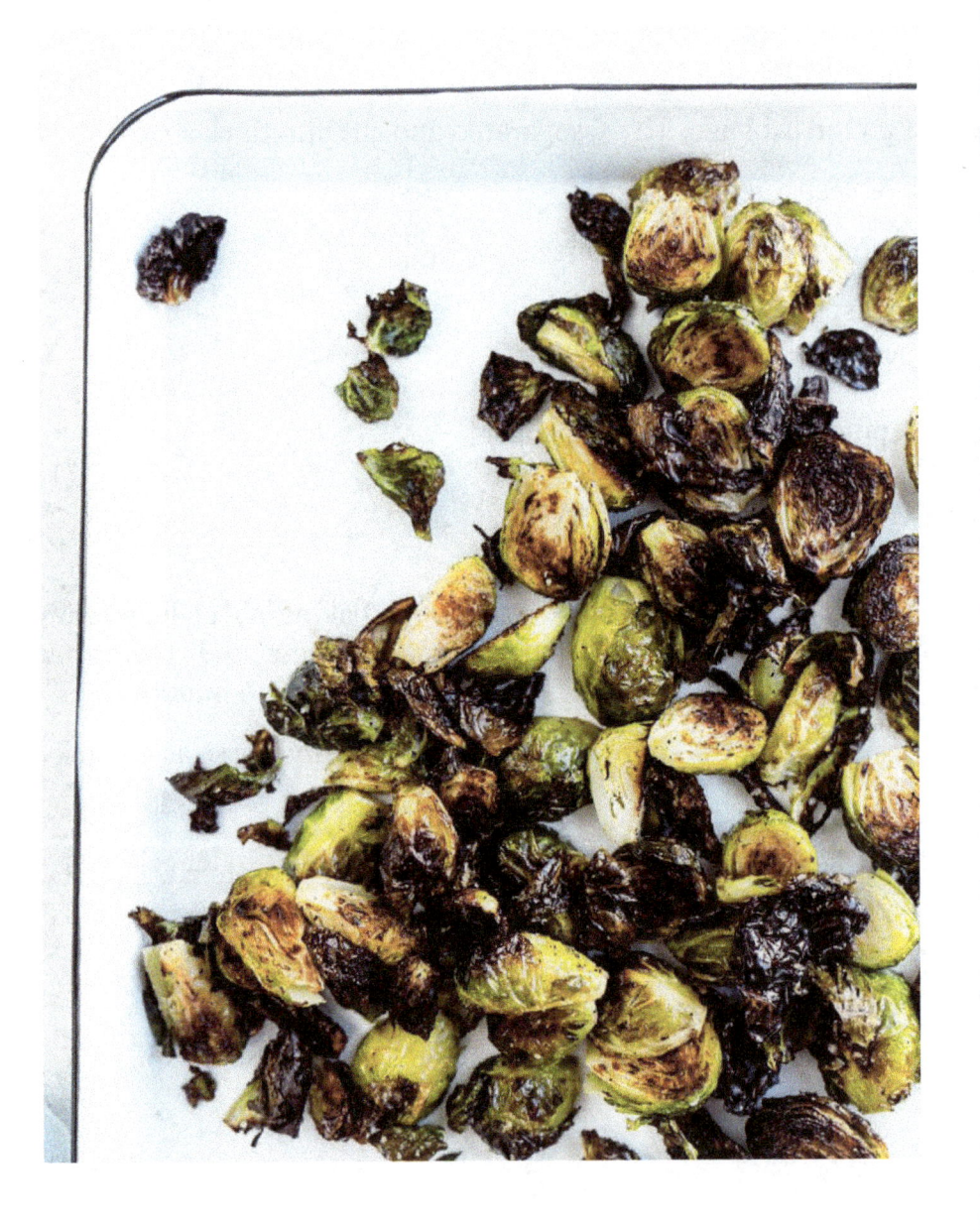

Preparation time: 10 minutes Cooking time: 30 minutes Servings: 4

Ingredients:

2 pounds Brussels sprouts, trimmed and halved

1 teaspoon red pepper flakes

1 tablespoon smoked paprika

2 tablespoons avocado oil

1 tablespoon balsamic vinegar

A pinch of salt and black pepper

Directions:

1. In a roasting pan, combine the sprouts with the pepper flakes, paprika and the other ingredients, toss and cook at 400 degrees F for 30 minutes.

2. Divide the Brussels sprouts into bowls and serve as a snack.

Nutrition: calories 162, fat 4, fiber 3, carbs 7, protein 8

Arugula Dip

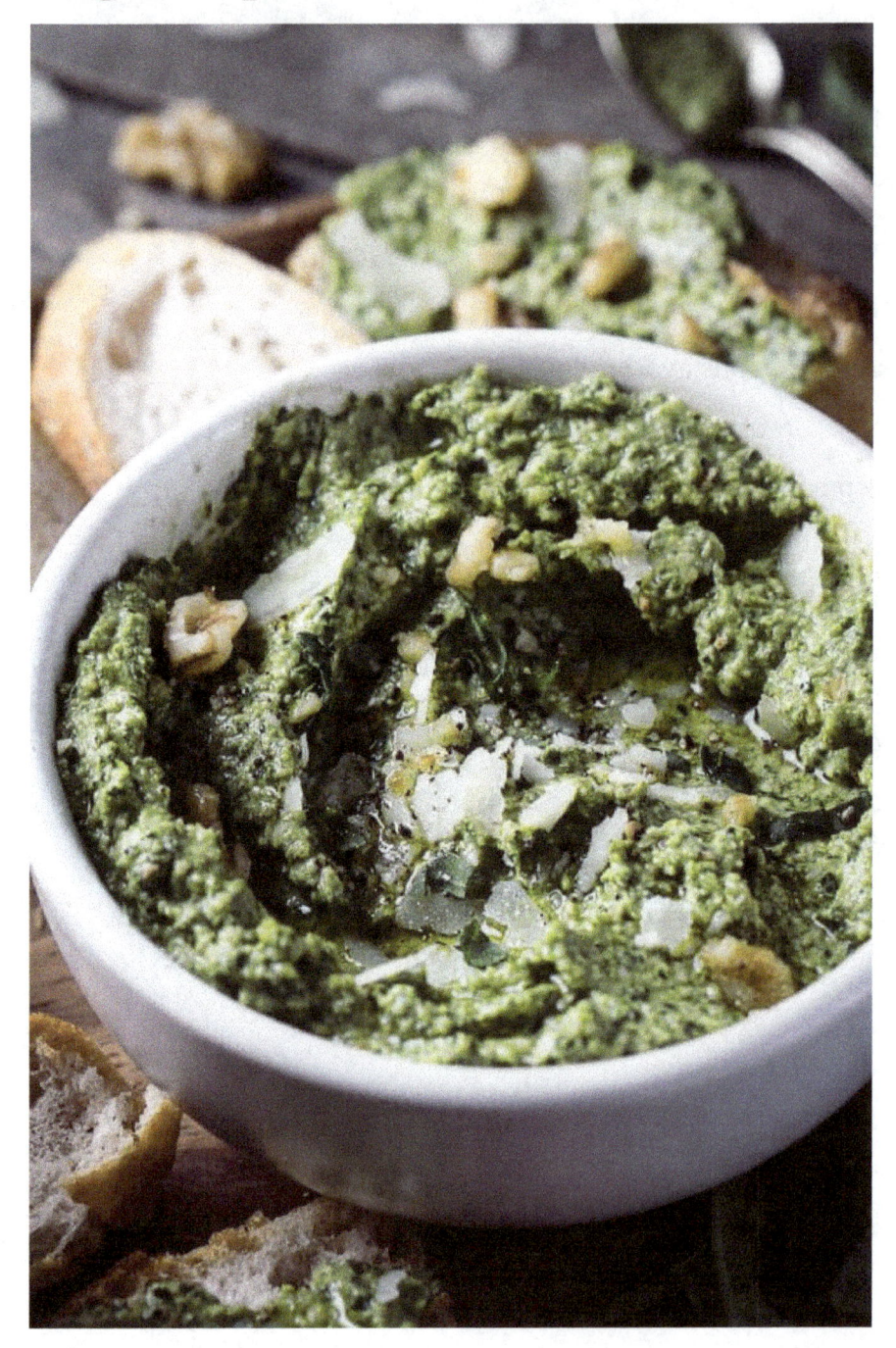

Preparation time: 10 minutes Cooking time: 0 minutes Servings: 4

Ingredients:

½ cup coconut cream

2 cups baby arugula

Juice of 1 lime

2 tablespoons walnuts, chopped

2 tablespoons olive oil

A pinch of salt and black pepper

2 garlic cloves minced

¼ teaspoon red pepper flakes, crushed

Directions:

1. In a blender, combine the arugula with the cream, lime juice and the other ingredients, pulse well, divide into bowls and serve as a party dip.

Nutrition: calories 100, fat 0, fiber 1, carbs 1, protein 3

Coconut Bites

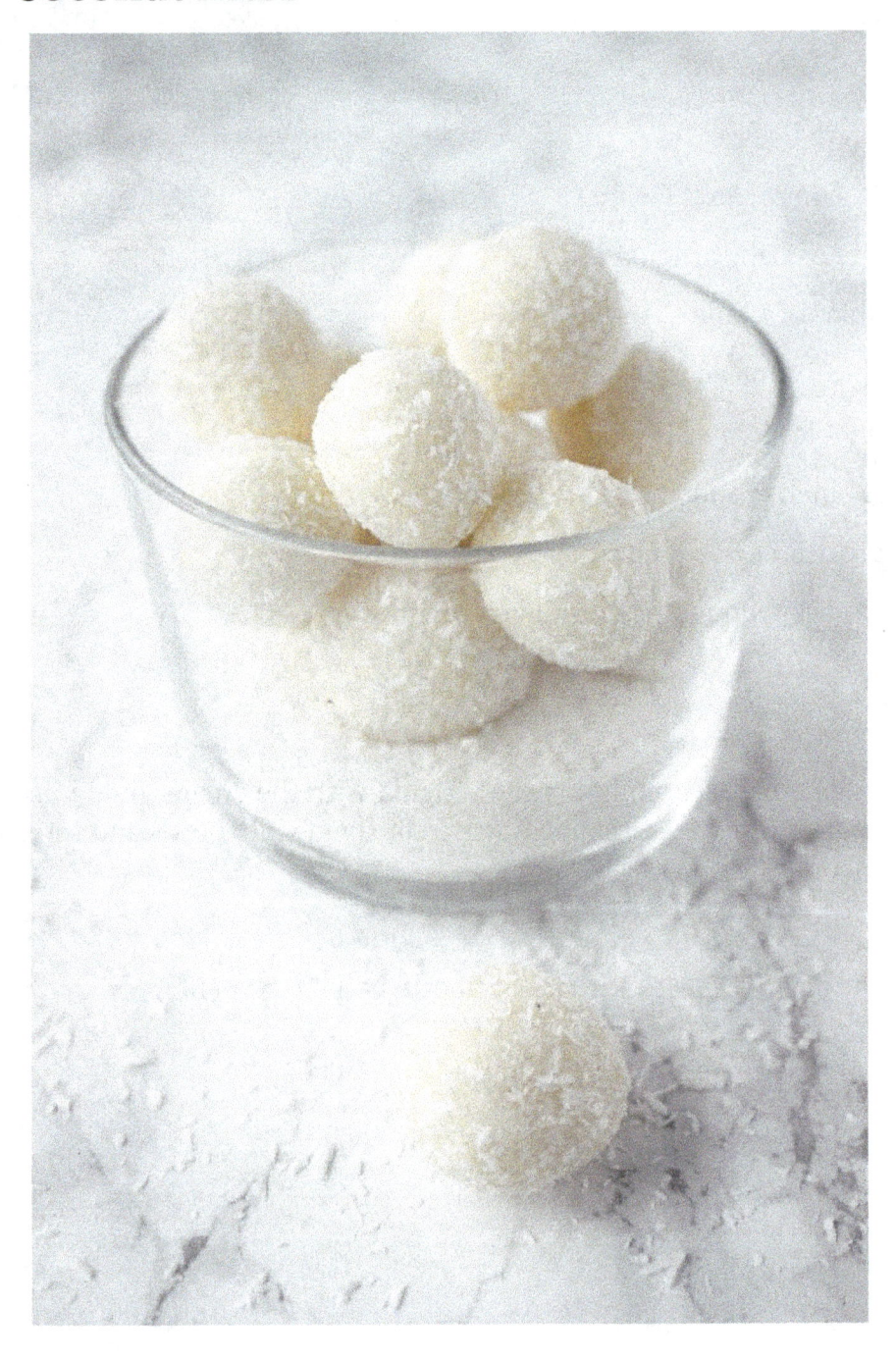

Preparation time: 10 minutes Cooking time: 25 minutes Servings: 6

Ingredients:

1 cup coconut milk

1 and ½ cup coconut flesh, unsweetened and shredded

A pinch of salt

¼ cup chives, chopped

2 teaspoons rosemary, dried

Cooking spray

Directions:

1. In a pan, combine the coconut with the coconut milk and the other ingredients except the cooking sp ray, whisk and cook over medium heat for 10 minutes.

2. Take spoonfuls of this mix, shape medium balls, arrange them all on a baking sheet lined with parchment paper, grease them with the cooking spray, and cook at 450 degrees F for 15 minutes.

3. Serve the coconut bites cold.

Nutrition: calories 112, fat 3, fiber 3, carbs 3, protein 8

Basil Eggplant Tapenade

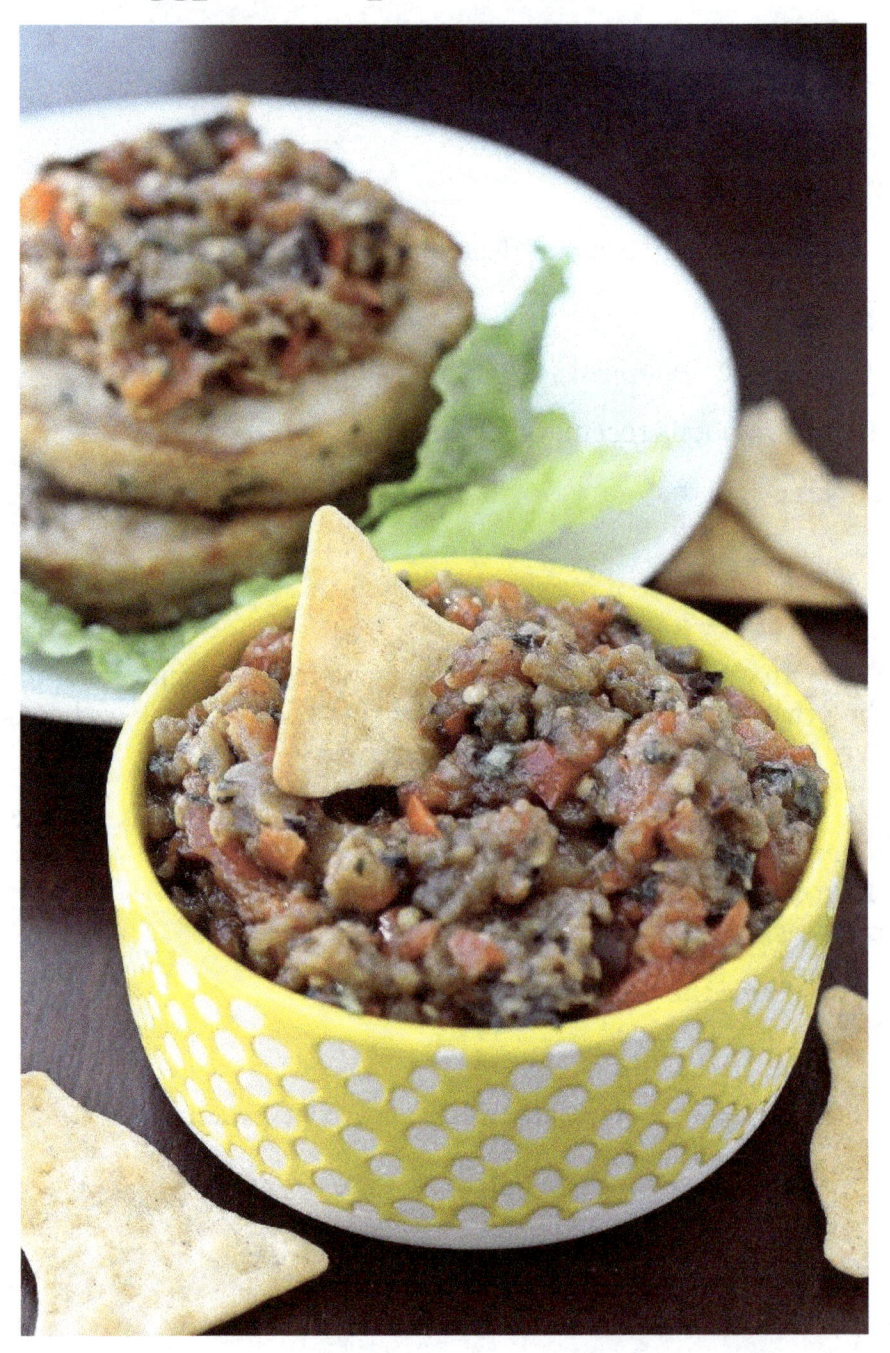

Preparation time: 10 minutes Cooking time: 15 minutes

Servings: 4

Ingredients:

1 cup cherry tomatoes, cubed

2 eggplants, cubed

2 tablespoons kalamata olives, pitted and cubed

1 avocado, peeled, pitted and cubed

2 tablespoons olive oil

3 garlic cloves, minced

2 teaspoons balsamic vinegar

1 tablespoon basil, chopped

A pinch of salt and black pepper

Directions:

1. Heat up a pan with the oil over medium heat, add the garlic, salt and pepper and sauté for 2 minutes.

2. Add the tomatoes, eggplants and the other ingredients, toss, cook over medium heat for 13 minutes, divide into small bowls and serve as an appetizer.

Nutrition: calories 121, fat 3, fiber 1, carbs 8, protein 12

Hot Eggplant and Broccoli Spread

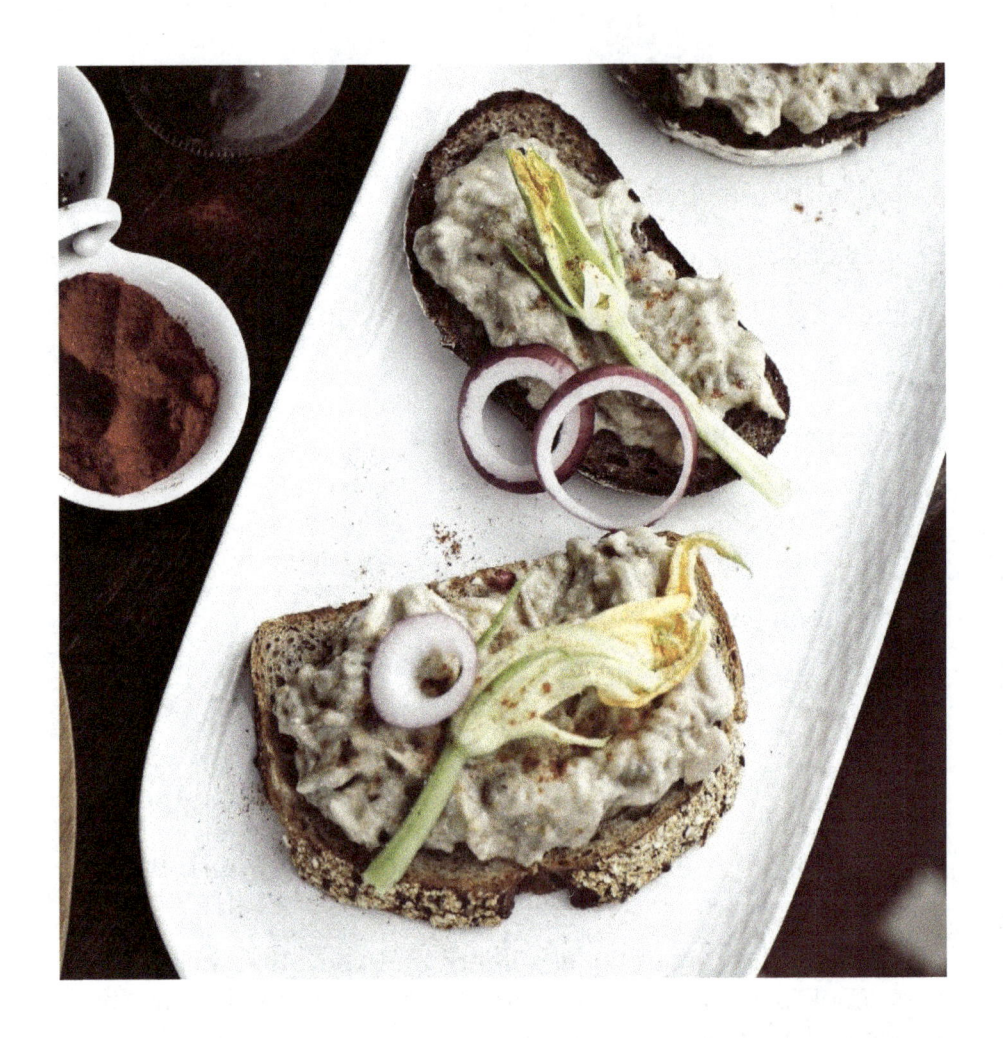

Preparation time: 10 minutes Cooking time: 25 minutes Servings: 8

Ingredients:

½ cup walnuts, chopped

2 eggplants, cubed

1 cup broccoli florets

1 cup coconut cream

1 teaspoon hot paprika

½ teaspoon chili powder

A pinch of salt and black pepper

½ teaspoon garlic powder

1 teaspoon cumin, ground

½ teaspoon rosemary, dried

Directions:

1. Heat up a pan with the cream over medium heat, add the walnuts, eggplants, broccoli and the other ingredients, stir, cook for 25 minutes and transfer to a blender.

2. Pulse well, divide into bowls and serve as a party spread.

Nutrition: calories 192, fat 5, fiber 7, carbs 9, protein 8

Almond and Pine Nuts Spread

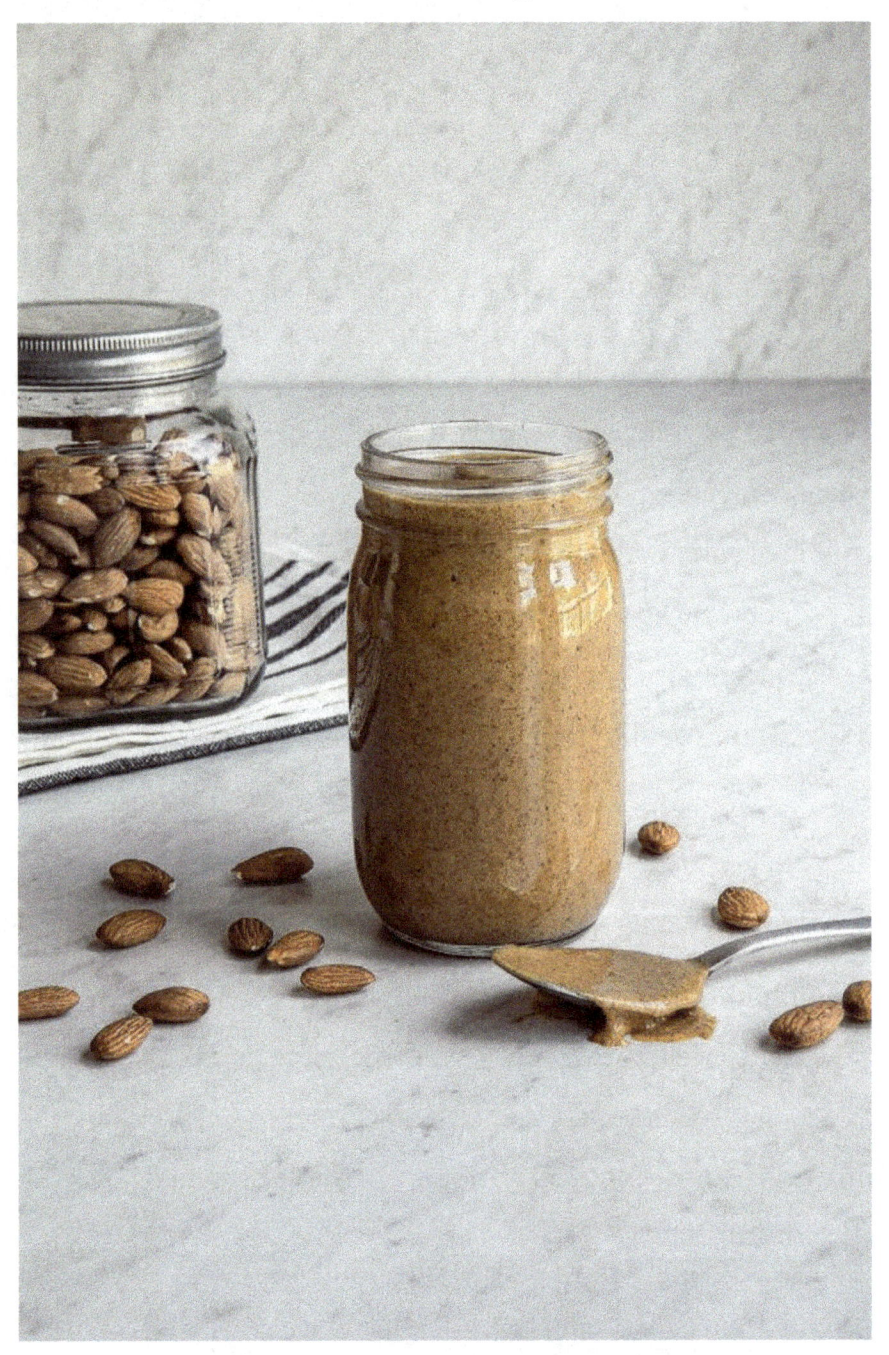

Preparation time: 10 minutes Cooking time: 15 minutes Servings: 8

Ingredients:

1 cup coconut cream

½ cup almonds, chopped

2 tablespoons pine nuts, toasted

1 tablespoon olive oil

1 teaspoon sage, ground

1 teaspoon chili powder

A pinch of salt and black pepper

Directions:

1. In a pot, combine the almonds with the pine nuts, cream and the other ingredients, stir, cook over medium heat for 15 minutes and transfer to a blender.

2. Pulse well, divide into bowls and serve as a party spread.

Nutrition: calories 112, fat 5, fiber 2, carbs 8, protein 10

Coconut Cashew Dip

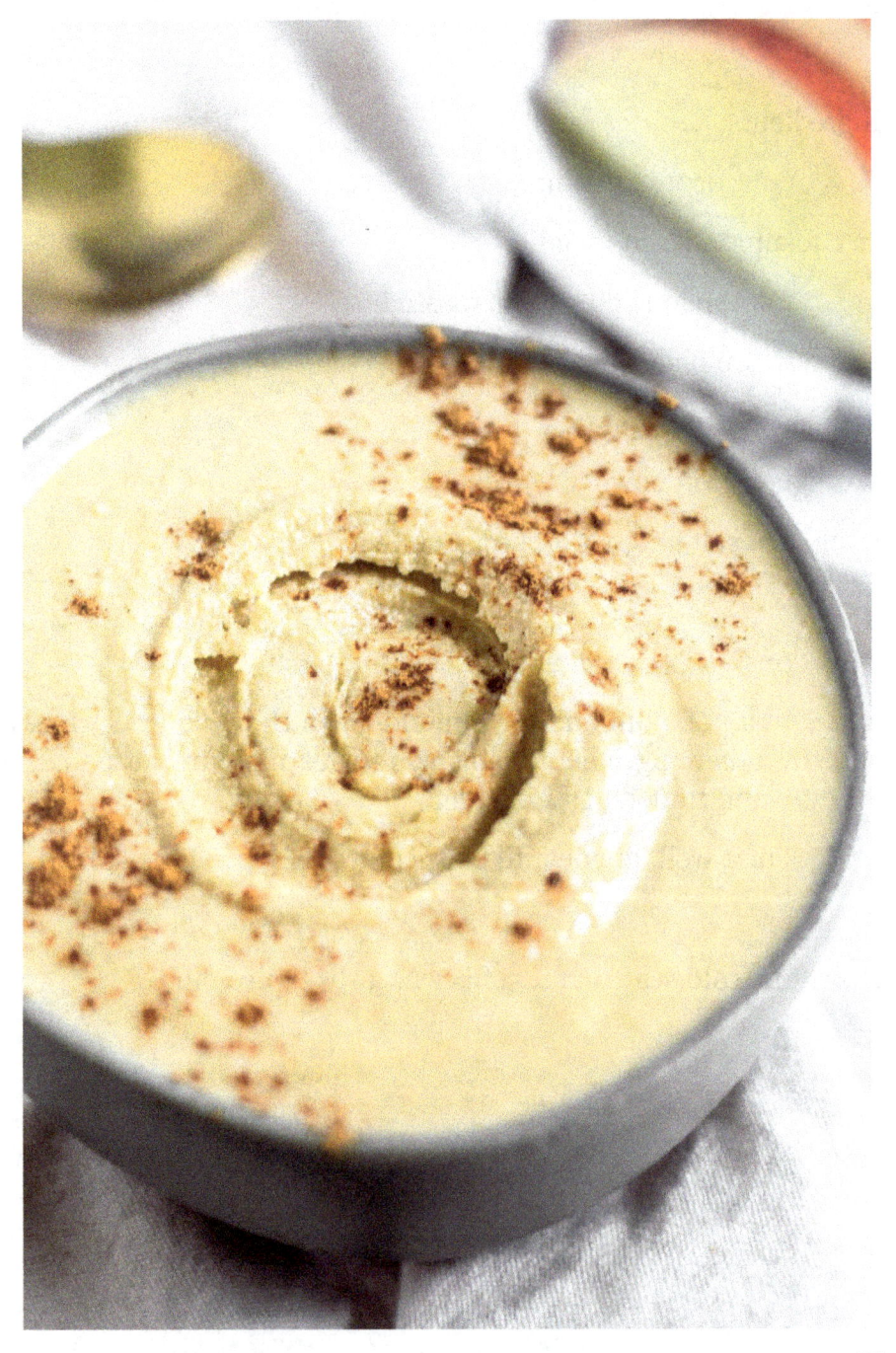

Preparation time: 10 minutes Cooking time: 30 minutes Servings: 4

Ingredients:

½ cup coconut cream

1	cup cashews, chopped

2	tablespoons cashew cheese, shredded

1 teaspoon balsamic vinegar

1 tablespoon chives, chopped

A pinch of salt and black pepper

Directions:

1.	In a pot, combine the cream with the cashew, cashew cheese and the other ingredients, stir, cook over medium heat for 30 minutes and transfer to a blender.

2.	Pulse well, divide into bowls and serve.

Nutrition: calories 100, fat 2, fiber 1, carbs 6, protein 6

Green Beans Dip

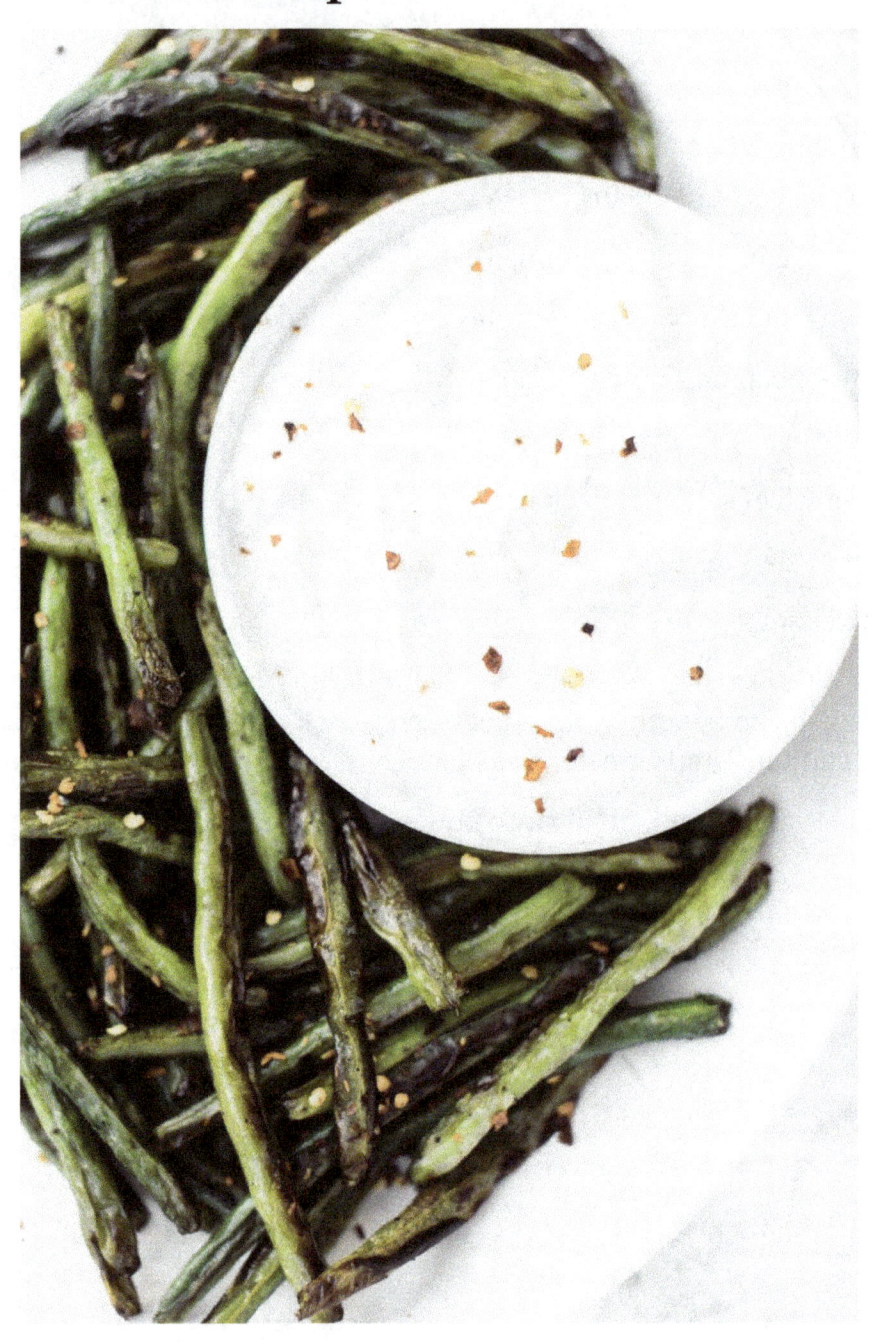

Preparation time: 10 minutes Cooking time: 25 minutes Servings: 4

Ingredients:

1 pound green beans, trimmed and halved

4 scallions, chopped

1 teaspoon turmeric powder

3 garlic cloves, minced

1 teaspoon rosemary, dried

1 and ½ cups coconut cream

A pinch of salt and black pepper

1 tablespoon chives, chopped

Directions:

1. In a pan, combine the green beans with the scallions, turmeric and the other ingredients, stir, cook over medium heat for 25 minutes and transfer to a bowl.

2. Blend the mix well, divide into bowls and serve as a party dip.

Nutrition: calories 172, fat 6, fiber 3, carbs 6, protein 8

Coriander Mint Chutney

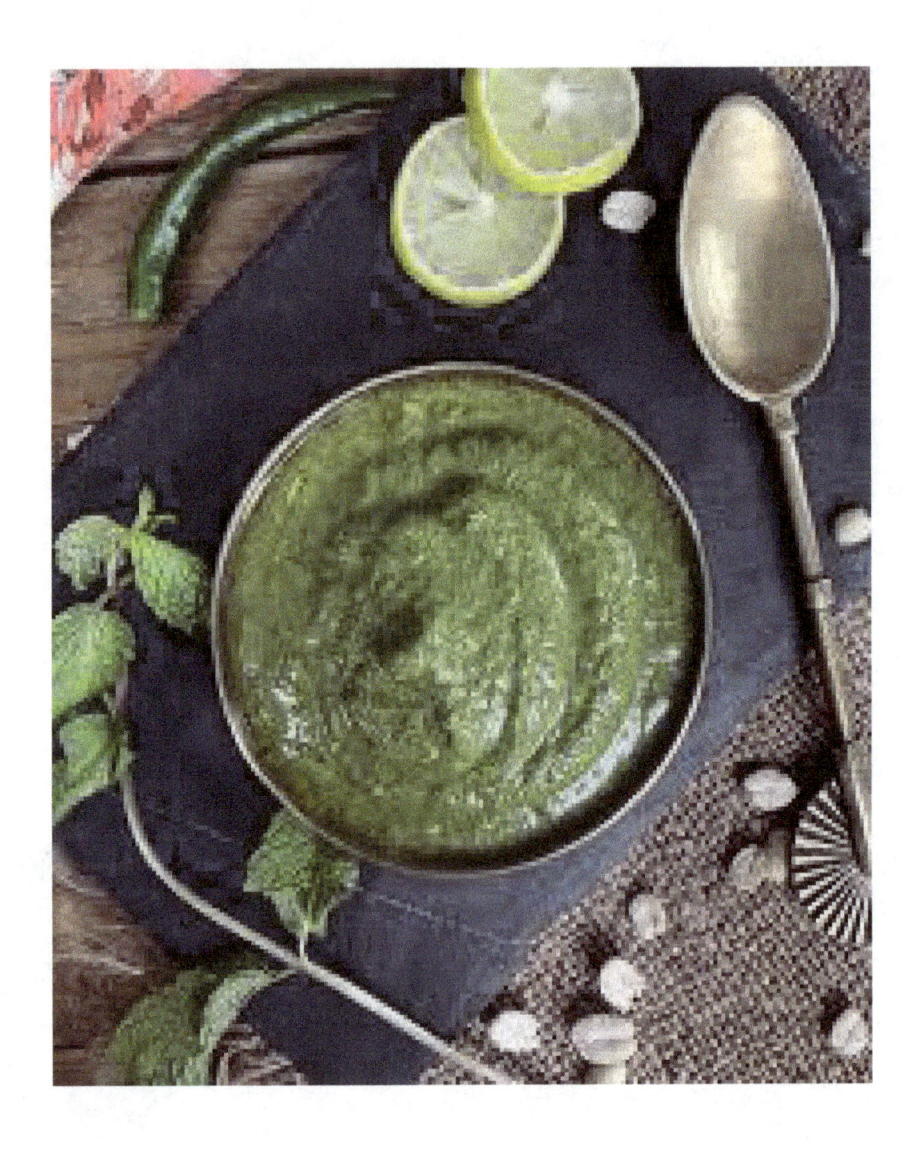

Preparation time: 10 minutes Cooking time: 12 minutes

Servings: 4

Ingredients:

1 and ½ teaspoons cumin seeds

1 and ½ teaspoons garam masala

½ teaspoon mustard seeds

2 tablespoons avocado oil

2 garlic cloves, minced

¼ cup veggie stock

1 cup mint

1 tablespoon ginger, grated

2 teaspoons lime juice

A pinch of salt and black pepper

Directions:

1. Heat up a pan with the oil over medium heat, add the cumin, garam masala, mustard seeds, garlic and ginger and cook for 5 minutes.

2. Add the mint and the other ingredients, stir, cook over medium heat for 7 minutes more, divide into bowls and serve as a snack.

Nutrition: calories 241, fat 4, fiber 7, carbs 10, protein 6

Spiced Okra Bites

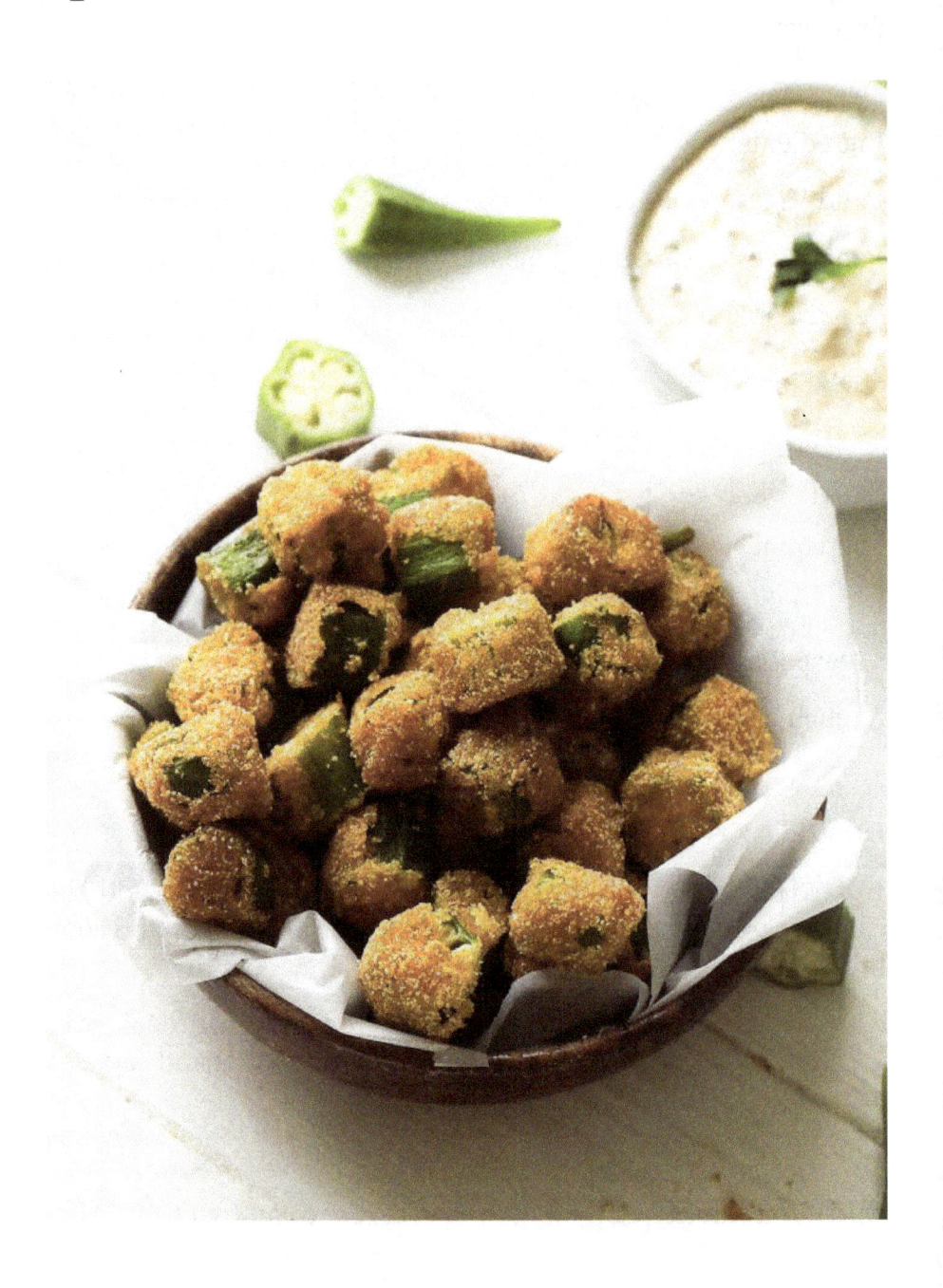

Preparation time: 10 minutes Cooking time: 15 minutes Servings: 4

Ingredients:

2 cups okra, sliced

2 tablespoons avocado oil

¼ teaspoon chili powder

¼ teaspoon mustard powder

¼ teaspoon garlic powder

¼ teaspoon onion powder

A pinch of salt and black pepper

Directions:

1. Spread the okra on a baking sheet lined with parchment paper, add the oil and the other ingredients, toss and roast at 400 degrees F for 15 minutes.

2. Divide the okra into bowls and serve as a snack.

Nutrition: calories 200, fat 2, fiber 2, carbs 6, protein 7

Rosemary Chard Dip

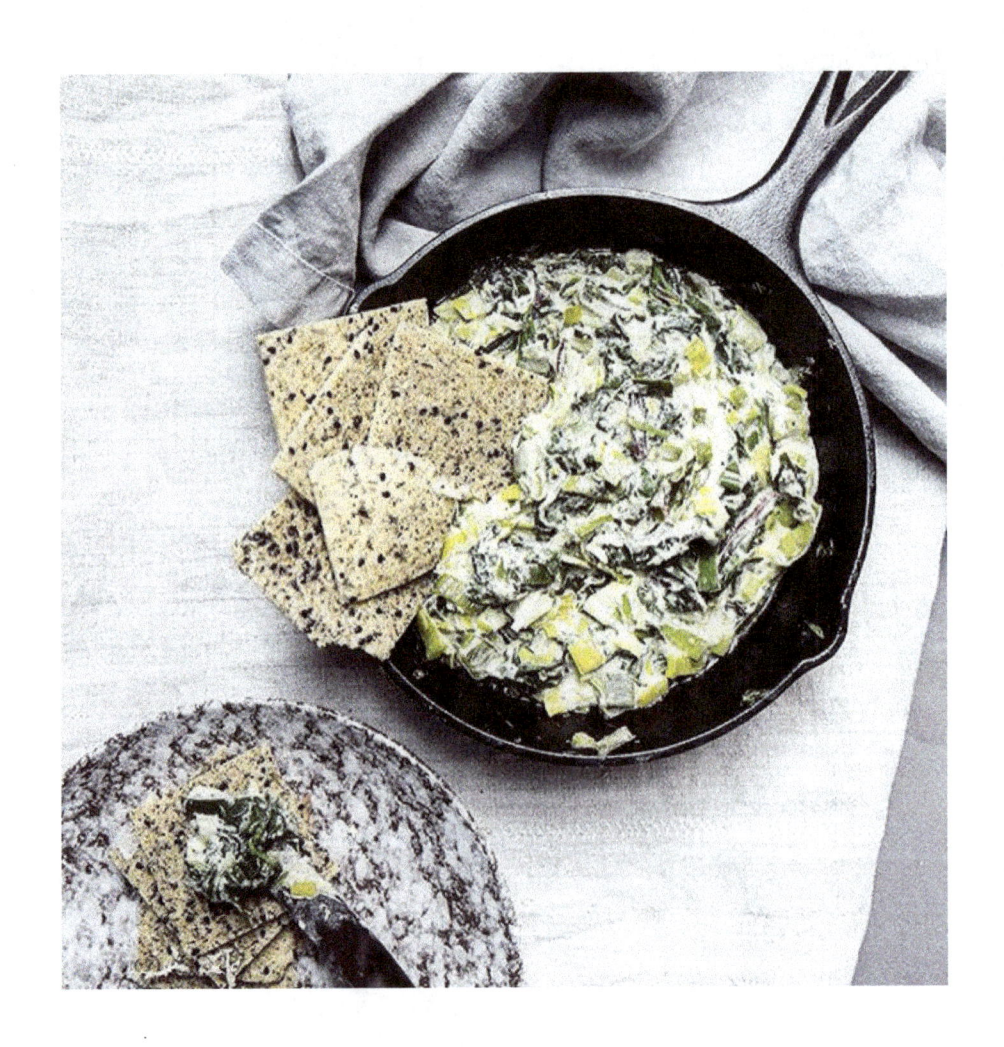

Preparation time: 10 minutes Cooking time: 20 minutes Servings: 4

Ingredients:

4 cups chard, chopped

2 cups coconut cream

½ cup cashews, chopped

A pinch of salt and black pepper

1 teaspoon smoked paprika

½ teaspoon chili powder

¼ teaspoon mustard powder

½ cup cilantro, chopped

Directions:

1. In a pan, combine the chard with the cream, cashews and the other ingredients, stir, cook over medium heat for 20 minutes and transfer to a blender.

2. Pulse well, divide into bowls and serve as a party dip.

Nutrition: calories 200, fat 4, fiber 3, carbs 6, protein 7

Spinach and Chard Hummus

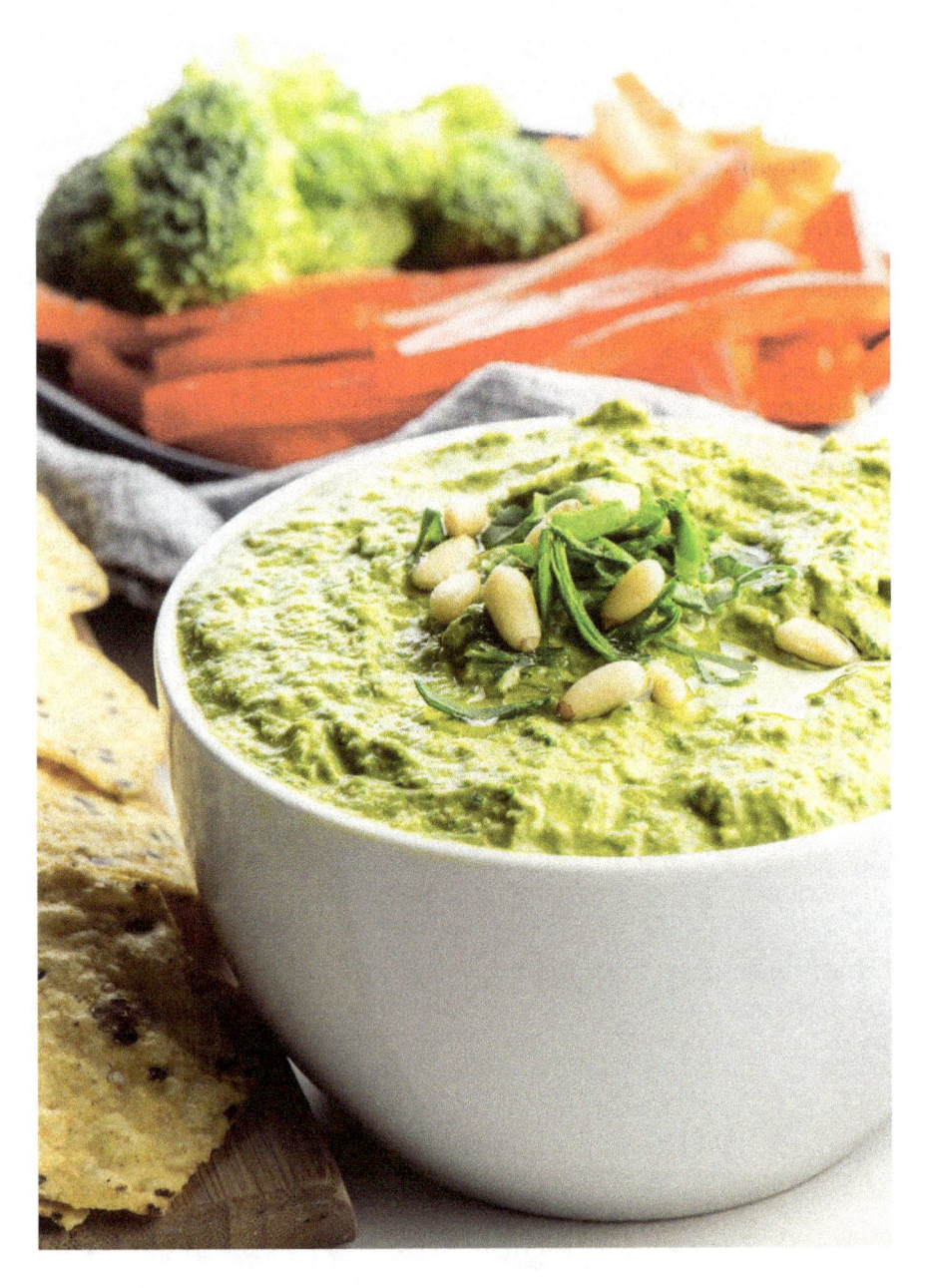

Preparation time: 10 minutes Cooking time: 10 minutes Servings: 4

Ingredients:

2 garlic cloves, minced

2 cup chard leaves

2 cups baby spinach

½ cup coconut cream

¼ cup sesame paste

A pinch of salt and black pepper

2 tablespoons olive oil

Juice of ½ lemon

Directions:

1. Put the cream in a pan, heat it up over medium heat, add the chard, garlic and the other ingredients, stir, cook for 10 minutes, blend using an immersion blender, divide into bowls and serve.

Nutrition: calories 172, fat 4, fiber 3, carbs 7, protein 8

Veggie Spread

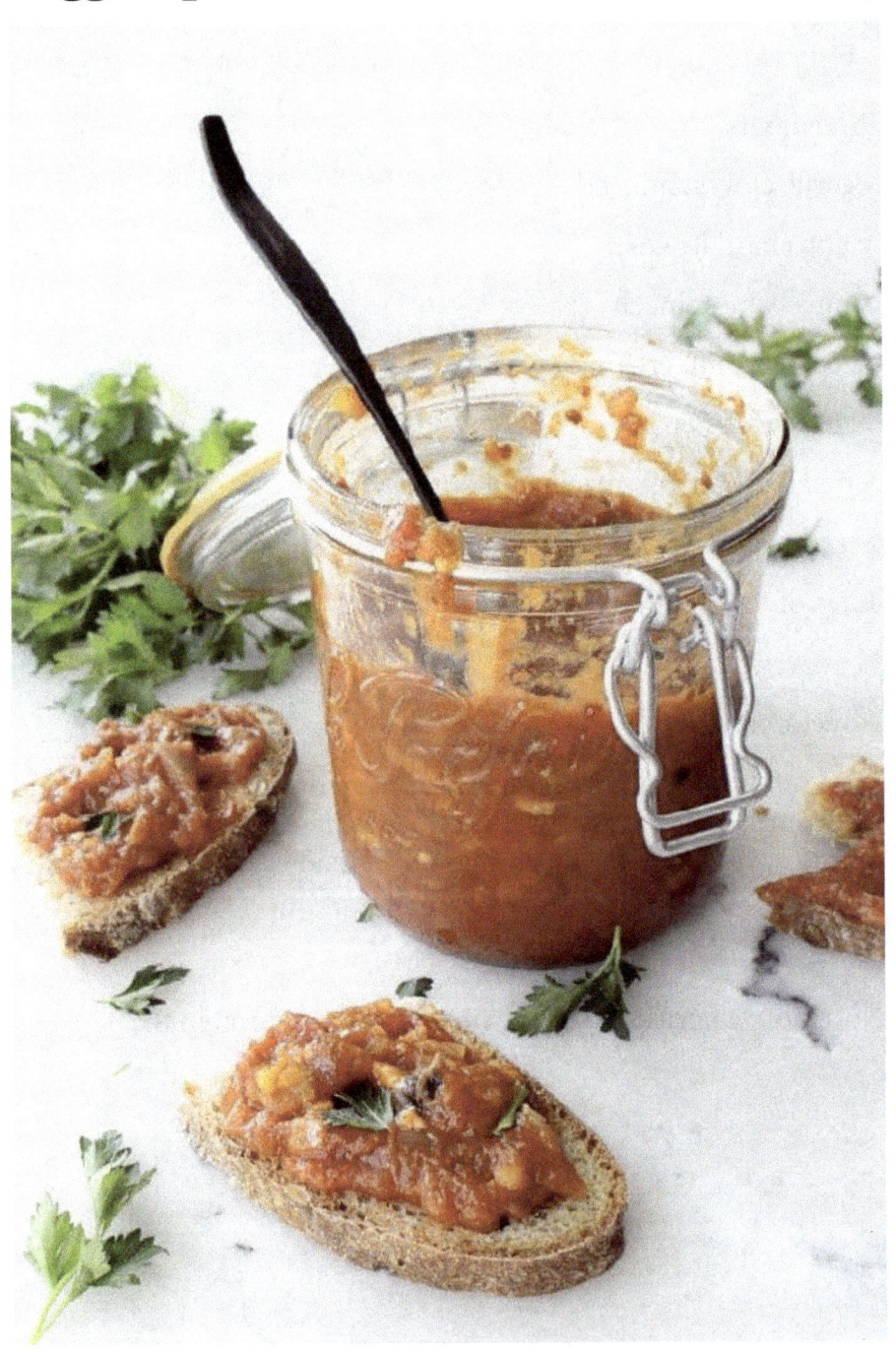

Preparation time: 10 minutes Cooking time: 20 minutes Servings: 4

Ingredients:

2 tablespoons olive oil

1 cup shallots, chopped

2 garlic cloves, minced

½ cup eggplant, chopped

½ cup red bell pepper, chopped

¼ cup tomatoes, cubed

2 tablespoons coconut cream

¼ cup veggie stock

Salt and black pepper to the taste

Directions:

1. Heat up a pan with the oil over medium heat, add the shallots and the garlic and sauté for 5 minutes.

2. Add the eggplant, tomatoes and the other ingredients, stir and cook for 15 minutes more.

3. Blend the mix a bit with an immersion blender, divide into bowls and serve cold as a party spread.

Nutrition: calories 163, fat 4, fiber 3, carbs 7, protein 8

Pomegranate Dip

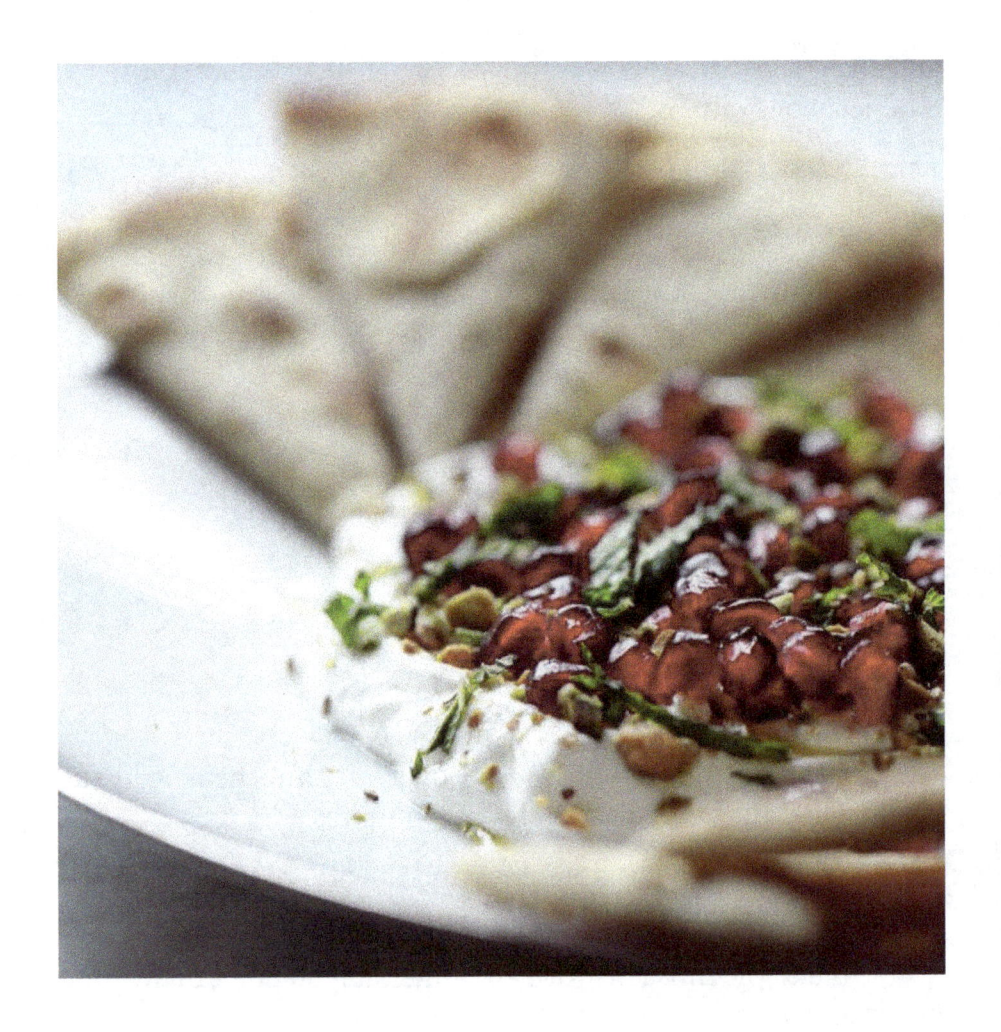

Preparation time: 10 minutes Cooking time: 0 minutes Servings: 6

Ingredients:

2 cups coconut cream

2 tablespoons walnuts, chopped

½ cup pomegranate seeds

A pinch of salt and white pepper

2 tablespoons mint, chopped

2 tablespoons olive oil

Directions:

1. In a blender, combine the cream with the pomegranate seeds and the other ingredients, pulse well, divide into bowls and serve cold.

Nutrition: calories 294, fat 18, fiber 1, carbs 21, protein 10

Tomato and Watermelon Bites

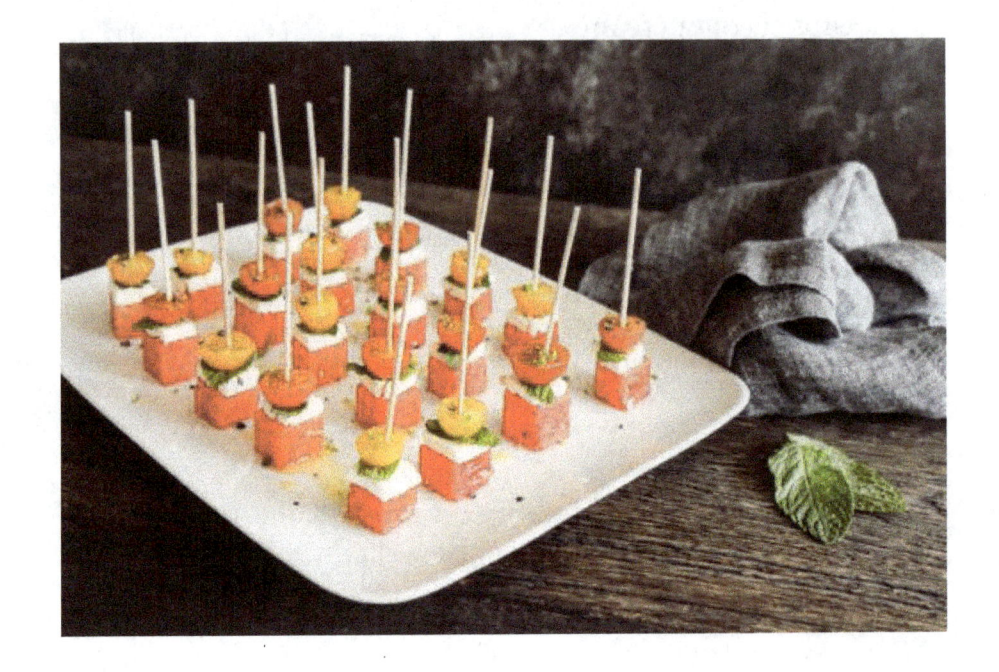

Preparation time: 10 minutes Cooking time: 0 minutes Servings: 6

Ingredients:

1/3 cup basil, chopped

1 pound cherry tomatoes, halved

2 cups watermelon, peeled and roughly cubed

1 teaspoon avocado oil

1 tablespoon balsamic vinegar

Directions:

1. In a bowl, combine the cherry tomatoes with the watermelon cubes and the other ingredients, toss, arrange on a platter and serve as an appetizer.

Nutrition: calories 162, fat 4 fiber 7, carbs 29, protein 4

Brown Betty Bananas Foster.

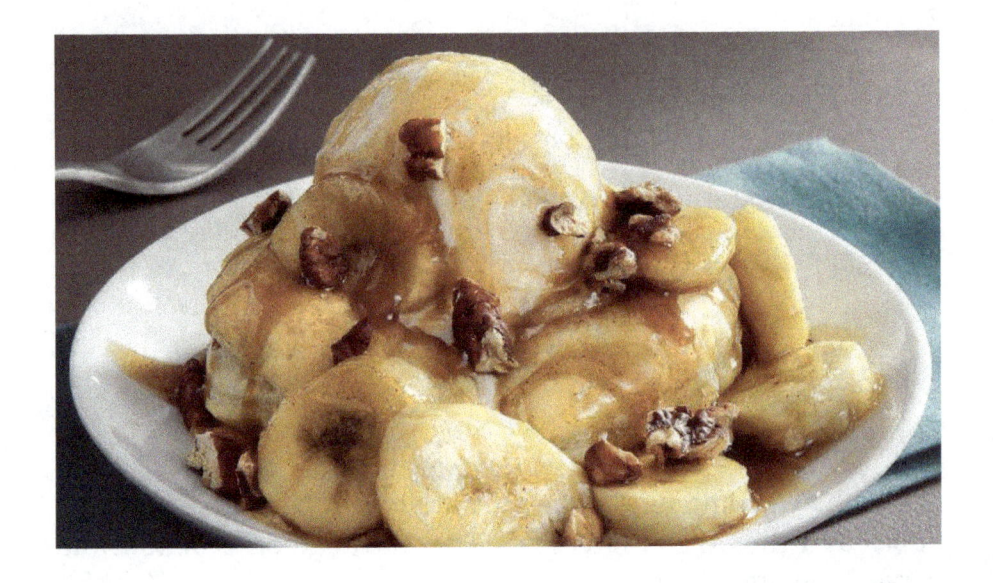

Preparation Time: 15 Minutes Servings: 4

Ingredients:

6 cups cubed white bread, a little stale helps

4 ripe bananas, peeled and chopped

⅓ cup chopped toasted pecans

⅓ cup pure maple syrup

⅓ cup packed light brown sugar or granulated natural sugar

¼ cup unsweetened almond milk

2 tablespoons brandy

½ teaspoon ground cinnamon

¼ teaspoon ground nutmeg

¼ teaspoon ground ginger

⅛ teaspoon salt

Directions:

1. Lightly oil a baking tray that will fit in the steamer basket of your Instant Pot.

2. In a bowl combine almond milk, maple syrup, and the spices.

3. Roll the bread cubes in the milk mix.

4. In another bowl mix the bananas, pecans, brandy, and sugar.

5. Layer your two mixes in the tray: half bread, half banana, half bread, half banana.

6. Pour the minimum amount of water into the base of your Instant Pot and lower the steamer basket.

7. Seal and cook on Steam for 12 minutes.

8. Release the pressure quickly and set to one side to cool a little.

Bread & Butter Pudding

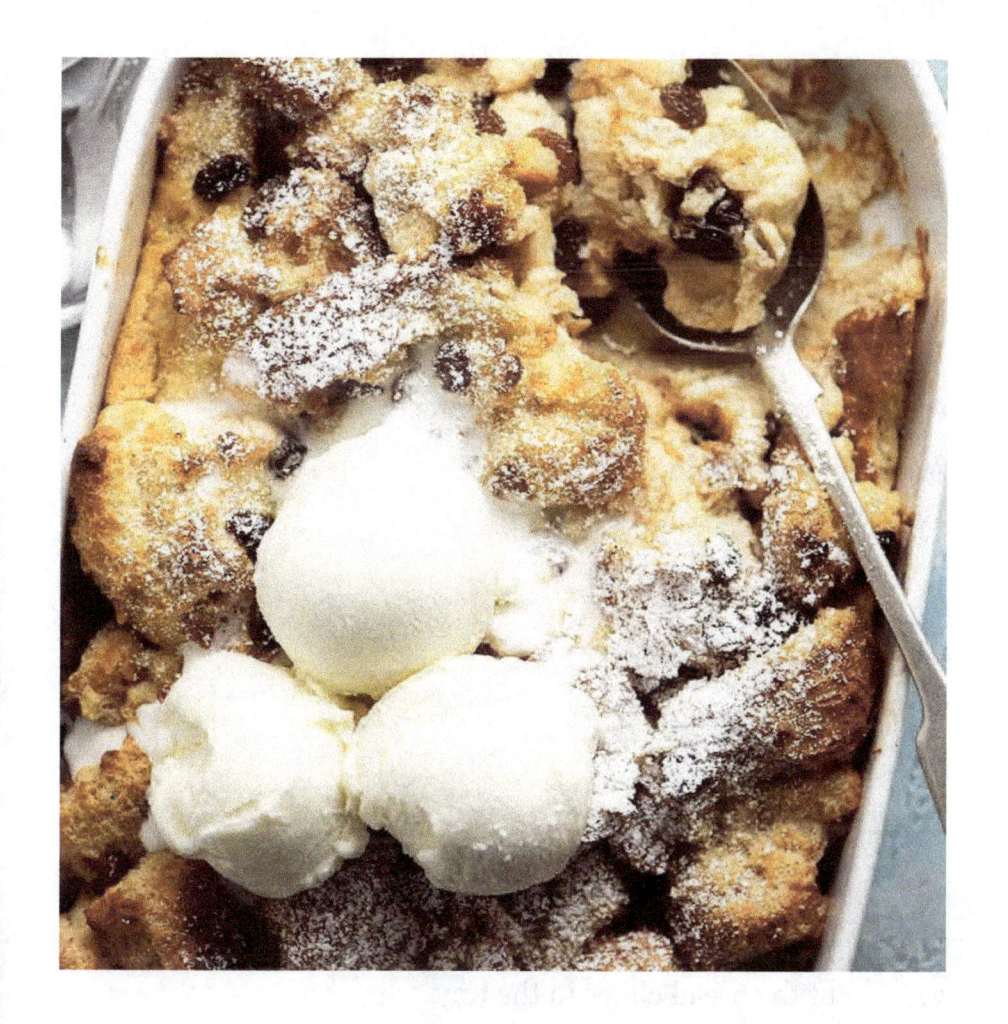

Preparation Time: 25 Minutes Servings: 8

Ingredients:

3 cups nondairy milk, warmed

2 cups cubed spiced bread or cake, stale is better

2 cups cubed whole-grain bread, stale is better

1 (16-ouncecan solid-pack pumpkin

¾ cup packed light brown sugar or granulated natural sugar

3 tablespoons rum or bourbon or 1 teaspoon rum extract (optional 1 teaspoon pure vanilla extract

1½ teaspoons ground cinnamon

¼ teaspoon ground nutmeg

¼ teaspoon ground allspice

¼ teaspoon ground ginger

¼ teaspoon salt

Directions:

1. Lightly oil a baking tray that will fit in the steamer basket of your Instant Pot.

2. Put the bread cubes in the tray.

3. Mix the pumpkin, sugar, vanilla, rum, spices, and salt.

4. Slowly stir in the milk.

5. Pour the mix over the bread.

6. Pour the minimum amount of water into the base of your Instant Pot and lower the steamer basket.

7. Seal and cook on Steam for 20 minutes.

8. Release the pressure quickly and set to one side to cool a little.

Custard Bread Pudding.

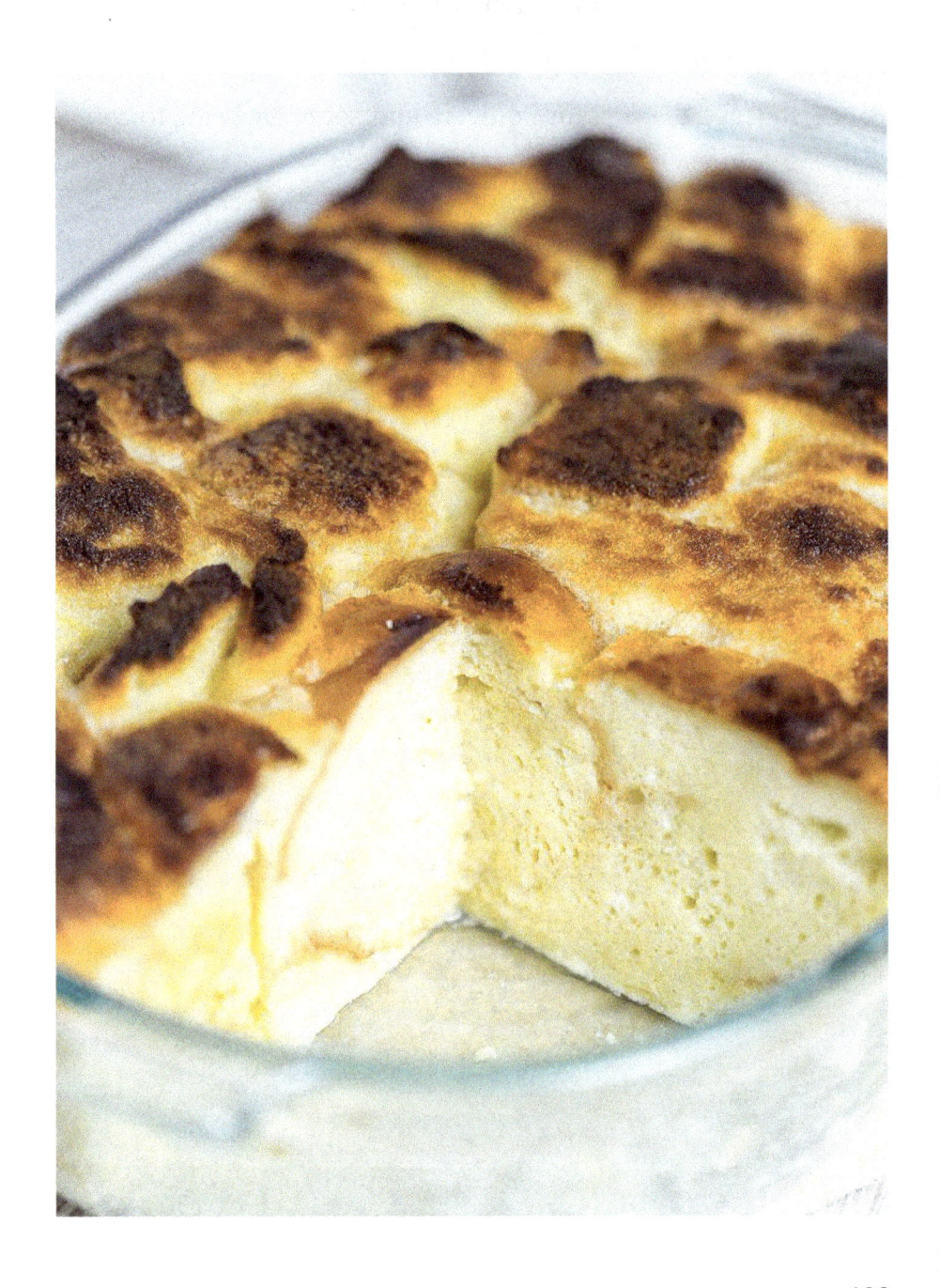

Preparation Time: 45 Minutes Servings: 6

Ingredients:

6 cups cubed white bread

3 cups unsweetened almond milk

2 cups fresh raspberries or sliced strawberries, for serving

½ cup vegan white chocolate chips

½ cup packed light brown sugar or granulated natural sugar

½ cup dry Marsala

Pinch of salt

Directions:

1. Melt your white chocolate into a cup of the almond milk. If using your Instant Pot, keep the lid off, stir throughout.
2. Add the Marsala, sugar, and salt.
3. Clean your Instant Pot.
4. Press half the bread cubes into the insert.
5. Pour half the Marsala mix on top.
6. Repeat.
7. Seal and cook on low for 35 minutes.
8. Release the pressure naturally.
9. Serve warm with fresh berries.

Warm Rum Butter Spiced Cider

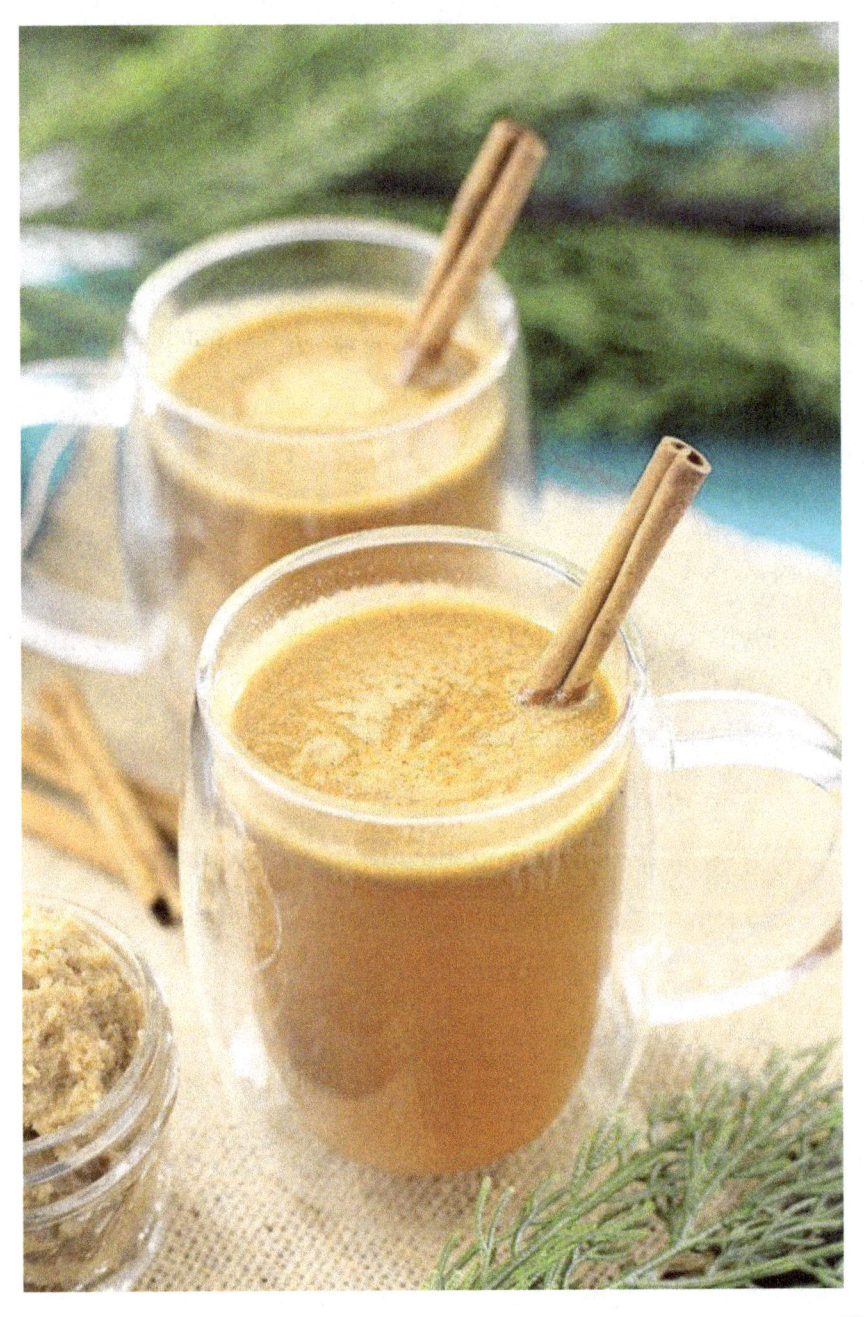

Preparation Time: 15 Minutes Servings: 4

Ingredients:

3/4 cup rum

4 cups apple cider

2 cinnamon sticks

4 cardamom pods

1/4 teaspoon ground allspice

4 whole cloves

1 teaspoon lime juice

4 teaspoons nondairy butter

Directions:

1. Combine all the ingredients in the instant pot. Seal the lid and cook on high 5 minutes. Let the pressure release naturally.